Spirituality, Ethics and Care

of related interest

Medicine of the Person
Faith, Science and Values in Health Care Provision
Edited by John Cox, Alastair V. Campbell and Bill K.W.M. Fulford
Foreword by Julia Neuberger
ISBN 978 1 84310 397 4

Making Sense of Spirituality in Nursing and Health Care Practice
An Interactive Approach
2nd edition
Wilfred McSherry
Foreword by Keith Cash
ISBN 978 1 84310 365 3

The Challenge of Practical Theology
Selected Essays
Stephen Pattison
ISBN 978 1 84310 453 7

Spirituality and Mental Health Care
Rediscovering a 'Forgotten' Dimension
John Swinton
ISBN 978 1 85302 804 5

Working Ethics
How to Be Fair in a Culturally Complex World
Richard Rowson
ISBN 978 1 85302 750 5

Spiritual Caregiving as Secular Sacrament
A Practical Theology for Professional Caregivers
Ray S. Anderson
Foreword by John Swinton
ISBN 978 1 84310 746 0

Spirituality in Health Care Contexts
Edited by Helen Orchard
ISBN 978 1 85302 969 1

Talking About Spirituality in Health Care Practice
A Resource for the Multi-Professional Health Care Team
Gillian White
ISBN 978 1 84310 305 9

Spirituality, Ethics and Care

Simon Robinson

Jessica Kingsley Publishers
London and Philadelphia

First published in 2008
by Jessica Kingsley Publishers
116 Pentonville Road
London N1 9JB, UK
and
400 Market Street, Suite 400
Philadelphia, PA 19106, USA

www.jkp.com

Library of Congress Cataloging in Publication Data
Robinson, Simon, 1951-
  Spirituality, ethics, and care / Simon Robinson.
      p. cm.
  Includes bibliographical references and index.
  ISBN 978-1-84310-498-8 (alk. paper)
  1. Religion and ethics. 2. Caring—Moral and ethical aspects. I. Title.
  BJ47.R58 2007
  205'.642—dc22
                                                          2007014675

British Library Cataloguing in Publication Data
A CIP catalogue record for this book is available from the British Library

ISBN 978 1 84310 498 8

Printed and bound in Great Britain by
Athenaeum Press, Gateshead, Tyne and Wear

This book has grown out of recent opportunities to do work on spirituality, ethics and professional practice at Leeds Metropolitan University, for which I have to thank the Vice-Chancellor Professor Simon Lee. Simon knows better than most how beliefs and values relate in professional practice and organizational development, and I dedicate this book, with all its faults, to him.

Contents

Introduction

This is a book that attempts to make connections. I have been concerned over the past decade with spirituality and health and social care, and with the development of moral meaning in pastoral care. On the face of it, there must be strong connections between moral meaning and spirituality. However, this is not often reflected in the health- and social-care literature. In health-care writings – and even more in medicine – there is little attempt to bring them together. Often spirituality is seen as being the same as religion, and religion is seen to be quite independent of ethical decision-making, unless you happen to be working with a patient or carer who wishes to assert their religious rights. Health and social-care ethics, on the other hand, tend to focus on particular areas of ethical concern, without any thought of how these might connect with spiritual meaning and practice. Such areas are for religious 'club members' only, so the implicit argument goes, not for practitioners in general. As in other areas of applied ethics, the tendency is for authors to nod their heads in the first section of their books at the different theories of ethics and then to leave them swiftly behind for the safety of issues and cases – entirely ignoring the even riskier waters of underlying values and belief systems.

When we turn to theology, ethics tends to emerge from theological paradigms, leaving unanswered the question of how theology relates to spirituality, and how that relates to ethics. Feminist ethics and pastoral theology has encouraged theologians to look beyond an assumed cognitive connection, stressing the importance of the affective domain. However, even here the connection with spirituality is not always clarified. A parallel dynamic is there in philosophy, particularly with neo-Aristotelian philosophers such as McIntyre (1981) stressing the importance of virtue and community. Such an ethic focuses on the reflection on purpose and practice and how these relate to character and identity. However, there has been little attempt to relate virtues systemically to the affective domain, (for example, through an analysis of empathy) and still less to see how they relate to belief systems or related rituals.

The debates about postmodernity, with their stress on responsibility (particularly in semiotics) have interestingly opened up these areas for much clearer inspection, though still without explicitly making connections between belief systems and spirituality as such.

I suspect that this lack of connection is partly to do with 'turf wars' between academic disciplines or different professions. As Bender (2005) notes, modern academic disciplines have tended to view research data discretely, claiming it as their own. Increasingly, however, the need for collaboration in research is being seen as essential (Bender 2005, McLeish 2005). Moreover, writers such as Barnett (1994) and Williams (2005) identify a core, higher experience of reflection and learning that transcends discipline boundaries. Similarly, the experience of listening and responding to the call and demands of 'the other', whoever or whatever that may be, is something that can be informed by several disciplines but captured exclusively by none.

The aim of this book, then, is to develop a broader view of spirituality and explore how this relates to ethics. I will argue that spirituality is central to the development of ethical identity and that this, in turn, affects how we approach ethical decisions. This has an essentially practical focus, i.e. to enable the integration of spirituality and ethics in health- and social-care practice, in all caring professions. The domination of separate disciplines and professions in practice development can so easily lead to a fragmentation of professional practice, with ethics or spirituality seen as being essentially separate areas of professional expertise. This can have the effect of fragmenting the professional response, thus disempowering both the care professional and the patient or client as he or she tries to make sense of the illness experience and any ethical challenge this might bring.

From the perspective of Christian pastoral theology and ethics I would also hope that this book might contribute to underlying debates about spiritual and moral meaning and suggest more effective ways of relating these to care practice as a whole. Hence, whilst I hope that this book might be accessible to practitioners of all spiritual perspectives, I will on occasions make comments around Christian theology.

Chapter 1 will look at the background to this area, including traditional views of the relationship between spirituality and ethics, the ways in which the connection has broken down (not least with the decline of formal religions and the narrowing of the definition of ethics) and the various attempts to reconnect spirituality and ethics. It begins to develop a relationship between spirituality and ethics that involves consciousness, critical reflection and mutuality.

Chapter 2, based around a case study in health-care, will outline a view of broader spirituality that includes religion. It focuses on spirituality as: awareness of the other; the capacity to respond to the other; and the development of life-meaning around those relationships. Such meaning includes broad and generic understandings of purpose, faith, hope and care. For patients and practitioners, illness can raise questions about such meaning in many different ways.

Chapter 3 will focus on a case study and develop a framework of ethics that relates directly to the broader view of spirituality. This will involve four stages: the development of awareness; working with plurality in values and beliefs; negotiating responsibility; and enabling creative response. The chapter ends with a case study about conjoined twins.

Chapter 4 then examines more closely the nature of love and how it brings together care, spirituality and ethics. Chapter 5 begins to look at the spirituality of professional ethics in care focused around the ethos and virtues of the community of care. Chapter 6 considers the extension of that community to the patient or client, what the related virtues might be, and how they are developed. Here I argue that virtues cannot be the foundation for ethics, but are both the means and fruits of the care relationship.

Chapter 7 looks squarely at how religion and spirituality might be directly challenged in the caring context, and finally, Chapter 8 looks at how justice relates to spirituality, and sums up the normative basis of spirituality.

Throughout the book I will make use of case studies, which will cover situations such as end-of-life decisions, conjoined twins, heart conditions, social work, mental health, and emergency care. All are real cases that have been anonymized and used with permission.

I hope that this book will:

- enable care practitioners across all professions to be alive to the importance of spirituality in any ethical situation

- provide a practical framework for the professional to engage, where appropriate, with the spirituality of the patient or client

- provide the means of developing a richer view of patient autonomy and responsibility

- offer ways of reflecting on and developing the underlying spirituality of the professional, and how this will affect his or her ethical decision-making.

1

Ethics, Religion and Spirituality

Case Study

Over a hundred students were attending a workshop on professional ethics in health-care. The seminar spent some time enabling the students to develop a methodology of ethical decision-making. Small group work led on to a class methodology, and the tutor was putting the final touches to this in dialogue with the students. A part of this methodology was about the examination of underlying values, and how the professional might articulate and challenge such values. The tutor asked if anything else should be included in that section. From the back of the class came the response 'doctrine', expressed in a matter-of-fact tone. The tutor turned to see the familiar face of a Muslim student, and paused. How was he going to respond to this, and meet the outcomes of the session?

Running through his mind were several possible responses:

- 'That's interesting, but actually it's best to wait until the classes on spirituality and professional practice that come at the end of the year to raise that. Next question.'

- 'Doctrine refers to the theological underpinning of religions and is not really relevant to a consideration of ethical decision-making'.

- 'I fully respect your viewpoint as a Muslim but that is something that you need to address personally'.

None of these felt right pedagogically or conceptually, and so the tutor decided to respect the intervention and simply ask the student to clarify what he meant. The student responded by explaining that doctrine involved underlying beliefs about existence in this world and the next. Any ethical decision that he made as a professional practitioner would not just be informed in some way by those beliefs but would also have an effect upon him now or in the future.

A former president of the Christian Union (a strongly evangelical student group) immediately stood up to say that he, too, had a doctrine, and that this doctrine was important for him because it provided a transcendent dimension in his ethical decision-making. He explained this as providing an understanding of purpose that always helped him to stand back from the complexities of an ethical issue.

This led to an aggrieved response from another student who declared himself an atheist and argued that none of this was relevant to professional practice. Before the tutor could respond, another self-proclaimed atheist stood up, saying 'I disagree. I am also an atheist, but that doesn't mean that I can't have a doctrine. I have beliefs about life and about what it means to be a professional, and they frame what I value, and affect how I respond to any ethical need.'

By this time the neatly organized outcomes of this workshop had gone out of the window, and the tutor encouraged the students to explore how all this might have relevance to the client and their ethical decision-making.

Introduction

I make no apologies for beginning with the experience of students rather than practitioners. This anecdote suggests several things:

- Ethics is not an objective or neutral activity, but takes place in the context of beliefs about life. Sometimes these beliefs may not be explicitly articulated, sometimes they may be explicit belief systems, which may be articulated in religions.

- Ethical decision-making in lived experience involves making sense of any situation such that beliefs connect with practice. These students were keen to make connections rather than keep boundaries between practice and concepts, values and beliefs, and their personal and professional lives.

Pulling against such insights were the constraints that the tutor felt. These were pushing reflection into different directions:

- The fragmentation of learning, such that doctrine would be defined in terms of a discipline or area of interest, and be 'dealt with' later.

- Anxiety about expertise, or lack of it. Could a tutor trained in ethics be qualified to enable reflection on religion or spirituality?

- Anxiety about belief. The year 2006 saw major debates in Britain and around the world about religious hatred and how to respond to it in law. These raised important questions about what might cause offence to religious communities. No tutor wants to get him- or herself into a situation where this might happen. It is safer just to respect personal beliefs. But does respecting personal beliefs mean that we should treat those beliefs as essentially private and not open to challenge? The Muslim student was clearly saying that his belief bridged the gap between private and professional life, informing professional and public decisions. If this is true then how can we begin to handle that in professional practice and how can we enable the patient or client to explore the connections? To begin to make sense of this, I will review how these connections used to be seen, how perspectives have changed, and the attempts that have been made to reconnect them.

Religion and ethics

As Stanley Hauerwas suggests, the relationship between ethics and spirituality, viewed exclusively in religious terms, was originally firmly fixed (Hauerwas and Wells 2004). In Christian terms the connection was so obvious that there was no need to refer to 'Christian Ethics', as if these were separate from non-religious ethics. Frankena also suggests several ways in which religion and ethics related (1986):

- Religion provides a metaphysical base for ethics through providing doctrines that begin to define something about a present and ultimate reality. Present reality may be a view of humanity that informs practice. In Christian terms this has classically led to different schools of thought stressing the negative and positive view of humanity, or interdependence of humanity. All this may establish a set of human needs that inform ethical practice. Ultimately reality is very much what lies behind 'this world', in terms of divine creation and presence, and what might happen beyond this world, at the end of time.

- Religion provides motivation. This motivation might be positive or negative. The religious person, for instance, might be concerned above all to serve God, a relationship sustained through prayer. This commitment to the higher being then acts as a continual reminder to attend to ethics (Frankena 1986). The second motivation, expressed by the Muslim student above is the attempt to attain salvation. Salvation in this approach depends upon the person doing good. Expressed negatively this means avoiding damnation. Ritual can also reinforce motivation. This is a process of habitual actions that remind religious participants about the core meaning of their belief system and how it relates to practice. As ritual tends to be expressed in community it also reinforces motivation because the individual is encouraged by the presence of others.

- Religion provides an unconditional and transcendent perspective for ethics, taking us beyond narrow or self-interest. Behind this is the acceptance of human limitations, material and moral, ultimately expressed in the theology of sin, i.e. the view that we as human beings are in a state of sin and thus unable to be ethical without the support of God or a particular religion.

- Religion in terms of spiritual experience and ritual can provide an awareness that enables better moral practice. Typically, religious experience (in the sense of an experience of the numinous) heightens awareness. This can have the effect of heightening awareness of the self and others, and of the environment. This, in turn, contributes to the development of moral consciousness and an awareness of people, context and the related issues in any moral situation.

- The religious community can play an important part in the moral formation of a person. This is partly through modelling good practice in the ethos and practice of the community, and in and through the associated stories and texts of the community. This is also tied to the development of ethical identity and thus of the character and the virtues that might be central to community life. The gifts of the spirit set out by St Paul are a good example of such virtues (I Corinthians 12). That very idea of the gifts of the spirit suggests that virtues are not just learned by imitation of any model, but in and through the relationships in the community – something we will return to later.

This sense of connection between religion and ethics has remained not only in the religious communities but is also commented on by many writers in broader areas, such as education. Tate (in Beck 1999, p.23), for instance, quotes the then Archbishop of Canterbury, George Carey, as saying that since the Enlightenment we 'have been living off the legacy of a deep, residual belief in God. But as people move further away from that, they find it more difficult to give a substantial basis for why they should be good'. Tate then concludes that religious education should be a vital part of the curriculum, and that the development of children's spirituality is important 'as the origin of the will to do what is right' (Beck 1999, p.23).

Breakdown of old certainties

However, some might question Carey's connections in the light of the work of Plato, who suggests that ethics are by definition autonomous. Plato set this out in terms of a dilemma: is something good because God commands it or does God command it because it is good? (Plato 2002) Are there reasons for being ethical that are independent from God? Of course, this is only really a dilemma if you buy into a particular view of God's sovereignty, as a being who knows what is good and who insists that one conforms to this without any questions.

Nonetheless, the idea of the autonomy of ethics invites us to view ethics as a separate domain from religion – one concerned with developing an objective/neutral way of reasoning out ethical issues. Without some idea of reasoning independent from a divine being, it becomes hard to understand why one should act ethically. Such a rigid division between religion and ethics is reinforced by the Enlightenment and the view of humanity as rational autonomous beings, responsible for working out their own response to ethical dilemmas.

This focus on reason also led to the questioning of metaphysics – doctrines about what underlies reality, such as the nature and purpose of humanity, creation or God. Metaphysics cannot be validated in an empirical way and thus a valid ethics cannot rely upon any such view (Lovin 2005). This even extends to cosmologies. As Reynolds and Schofer (2005) note, in many religions cosmology is closely connected to ethics, with ideas of harmony between individuals, society and the cosmos, or views of the cosmos as essentially just or benign. Modern scientific cosmology, however, has been shorn of any ethical significance. Any basis of certainty for an ethical position has been further questioned by postmodern scholars who debate whether we are in so called postmodern times and, if so, how such a world might be characterized (Connor 1989). It is, however, possible to distinguish between postmodernism as theory and the experience of the postmodern era. In the first of these, new ways of understanding language and social constructs are argued for. Baudrillard (1983), for instance, sees the division between art and life as breaking down. There is no objective sense of reality and persons have to create their own reality and underlying life-meaning. Whether or not we agree with such theory it is hard not to accept something of our current postmodern *experience*, in which old certainties have indeed broken down. Our age is characterized by:

- An explosion of scientific and technological progress, making resources available that were undreamed of even fifty years ago. (The feminist movement, for instance, is unlikely to have grown in the way that it did without the technological means to sexual freedom, such as contraceptives.) At the same time this has led to a stress on rights and choice, often expressed in legislation, and also to new attitudes and value perspectives.

- An increasing influence of theories that stress relativity, indeterminacy or chaos. These began with Freud and his stress on the Unconscious, and culminated in postmodern thinkers such as Lyotard, Baudrillard and Derrida (Reader 1997). These French theorists, in particular, rejected any natural foundations to knowledge, or any correspondence between language and reality. Even the human person is no longer seen as autonomous, but rather the effect of discourse or power systems.

- A breakdown of patterns of behaviour and institutions such as marriage and the family, caused partly by the increase in wealth and increased mobility, but also by changes in attitude towards the sanctity of marriage and the idea of securing a partnership for life.

- A greater development and awareness of cultural and religious diversity within society, caused by increased migration and global awareness (Markham 1994). With this comes an acceptance of ethical plurality and, in turn, ethical relativity – the view that there can be no one basis of ethics.

All the above phenomena have combined to lead to a breakdown of any sense of objective knowledge and, in particular, adherence to the so-called 'grand narratives' that went before in the 19th and 20th centuries. Grand narratives are those stories that claim some universal truth (Lyotard 1979). They range from views about the person – characterized after the Enlightenment as autonomous rational decision-maker – to views about the purpose of humanity – dominated in the West by the Christian ethic. Such grand narratives might exist in the minds of the great thinkers or they might give meaning and purpose to whole nations that help to sustain them through times of crisis. The grand narrative of the British Empire, for instance, gave meaning to the people of Britain and beyond, undergirding the initial acceptance of the sacrifice of so many in the First World War. We no longer buy into those narratives in quite the same way since much of these cultural and economic underpinnings have disappeared. The major conflagrations of the First World War raised questions about the underlying assumptions it was fought for, leading eventually to a greater stress on individualism and the values of the free market. Lyotard (1979) argued that the grand narratives have now been replaced by many different narratives, both local and national. There are still some major narratives, including national loyalty, consumerism, the free market and the more communitarian views (with a stress on the importance on the development of community). However, these are now either in competition or dialogue (Brueggemann 1997). None of these narratives are more acceptable than the other and there are no privileged interpreters of any meaning.

With the advent of the so-called 'New Age Movement' polarity and autonomy were further stressed. Beginning in the 1960s, this was a loose collection of different movements and ideas that asserted many different spiritualities. They generated a real sense of excitement and inspiration focused on the idea that each person can discover, control and develop his or her own spirituality in their own way. A common theme throughout this movement is asserting freedom from a view of spirituality that had been imposed by patriarchal institutions and authorities.

Other central themes include:

- Any form of spirituality as being acceptable, whatever the form, unless it harms an other. Hence there is now a tolerance for a great range of spirituality. Indeed, all existence is seen as a manifestation of some greater Spirit and all religions are regarded as expressions of this same reality.

- Everyone is free to choose his or her own spiritual path.

- Spirituality as concerned with the 'other worldly', stressing the mystical and even magical. This seems a conscious attempt to locate spirituality in the numinous – that which is beyond and greater than oneself.

- Spirituality as largely anti-rational. Feelings and experience are paramount.

- All life is interconnected and human beings work together with the Spirit to create reality.

- At the source of all this, for some, is a form of cosmic love that enables all human beings to be responsible for themselves and for the Environment (Perry 1992).

Underlying much of this was a strong sense of the intrinsic goodness of humanity and a sense of a continued evolution towards spiritual enlightenment, both for the individual and the community. Whilst there is some sense of novelty about this movement it is also concerned with recapturing something of the past. Hence, paganism, for example, claims a history extending back well before the Christian era (Perry 1992). Many New Age groups are also concerned to chart the connection between spirituality and well-being and health, leading to a proliferation of complementary therapies (Watt 1985).

However, the New Age Movement is not without its critics. Its optimism about human nature and society, for instance, has little sustained empirical support. Since the flowering of the movement, there have been many examples of conflict and disasters – in the Middle East, the Balkans, Southern Africa, and so on – which do not indicate spiritual evolution. Second, the movement, by definition, lacks critical rigour. If all forms of spirituality are acceptable then there can be no common criteria for how to judge the claims and the worth of any particular spirituality. Third, the movement is not as inclusive as it would claim. On the contrary, the majority of New Agers are, in fact, articulate, middle-class and middle-aged. They have no more success in connecting with the vast majority of the population than do the main-line faiths (Perry 1995).

Nonetheless, the New Age Movement remains important to any understanding of spirituality in the West in recent years. Perry sums it up in this way:

> In general…it demonstrates a high degree of social and ecological awareness; it demonstrates a particularly useful attitude in understanding that life can be led as a self reflective process of growth and transformation; and liberates spirituality from the confines of religious dogma and empowers direct personal experience. (p.36)

Spirituality, ethics and health-care

Postmodernity and the New Age have raised questions about the nature of religion and challenged its place in society, further querying why religion should be the basis of ethics. Meanwhile, within health-care there has been an increased focus on spirituality as part of the therapeutic response, especially in the nursing profession. There are several reasons for this:

- First, a good deal of the history of nursing is based in some understanding of spirituality (Bradshaw 1994).

- Second, the concern for holistic care evidenced in recent years inevitably seeks to include all aspects of care. Indeed, for many, holistic care is tantamount to spirituality, connecting mind, body, and spirit (Papadopoulos 1999).

- Third, there is increasing research confirming a positive relation between spirituality and well-being, and thus successful therapy (Miller 2003a).

- Fourth, the nurse, in general, spends more time with the patient than do other health-care professionals, and thus can actually get to know the patient better than doctor or chaplain. Hence, some argue that spiritual care is integral to the role of the care professional, not just to clergy or chaplains (O'Brien 1998).

This concern for spiritual care is also 'driven' through a number of professional codes or educational recommendations. In nursing, there is a recommendation in one of its codes that nurses should be able to 'Undertake and document a comprehensive, systematic and accurate nursing assessment of physiological, social and spiritual needs of patients, clients and communities' (UKCC 2000, p.13). The American Association of Colleges of Nursing takes this a stage further. The nurse should be able to 'Comprehend the meaning of human spirituality in order to recognise the relationship of beliefs to culture, behaviour, health and healing… and to plan and implement this care' (AACN 1986, p.5).

Such approaches were reinforced by the revised Patient's Charter which assured the patient that, 'NHS staff will respect your privacy and dignity. They will be sensitive to and respect your religious, spiritual and cultural needs at all times' (DOH 2001, p.29).

There are, however, no guidelines on how these aims might be achieved. Moreover, within the different references there seem to be different emphases. Some see religion as being the same as spirituality. Others, such as the Patient's Charter, can distinguish religious from spiritual needs, though do not say what the distinction is. In some ways the most interesting is the AACN code. This looks at the way in which beliefs, not simply religious ones, relate to different aspects of the patient's life-meaning and experience. Intriguing though this is, however, there are again no indications of how such comprehension might be achieved.

It is perhaps not surprising that in nursing the actual practice of spiritual care is very variable (Oldnall 1996). The very different approaches and the lack of clear direction about the nature of spirituality also reveal a lack of clear aims and objectives in health-care training, and difficulty in determining how the different professions might work together around this theme. Nonetheless, there has been increased research into the nature of spirituality in health and health-care, not least into the definition of spiritual needs in illness (Robinson, Kendrick and Brown 2003).

The effect of all this in terms of professional practice has been to lay claim to a broader, practice-centred spirituality, but also to further decouple spirituality from ethics:

- The focus of practice has been on spirituality and therapy – how spirituality relates and contributes to recovery and well-being.

- Religion has increasingly been seen publicly in terms of fulfilling rights, something reinforced by employment legislation on religious rights (Employment Equality [Religion or Belief] Regulations 2003). As such, the connection between faith and ethics has not been explored.

- Ethics has also focused on the right of the person to decide, and the broader view of spirituality on autonomy from organized religion, and the right of the person to believe what he or she wants. This, in turn, has discouraged the development of shared vocabulary about spirituality and ethics or the development of any safe place for reflecting about such ideas. The result has been to make ethics and spirituality private. In one sense the 'privatizing' had already begun. The power structures of the churches tended to discourage reflection within churches, seeing the priest or minister as the 'expert' or 'guru' who embodied the orthodoxy and spoke for the community. This is well demonstrated by Hull (1991) in relation to religious attitudes that have discouraged learning. Such a dynamic is reinforced by elements in the postmodern world, with its stress on individual taste and a liberal view of freedom, as freedom from interference (Kendrick and Robinson 2002).

- Professionalization has tended to stress discrete areas of expertise, rather than connections. Hence, professional ethics and health-care has tended to focus on applied ethics (see Seedhouse 2002, Tschudin 2003). The model of applied ethics has assumed the autonomy of ethics, and focused on moral reasoning, and ethical methods, with little reference to any underlying cultural or religious meaning. Equally there has been little focus on the underlying meaning and purpose of the health-care professions, and hence on any ethical/ spiritual identity.

Building bridges

So, how can spirituality be reconnected to ethics? I will now examine several different attempts that have been made by philosophy, theology, religious ethics and the study of moral development.

Philosophy

Iris Murdoch, philosopher and novelist, had a strong sense of moral meaning as being connected to narrative and the development of identity. Her major philosophical works aim to break out of a narrow view of moral philosophy. As Taylor (1996) puts it, she argued against ethics as focusing on narrow views of obligation, i.e. 'what it is right to do' in any situation, and for ethics as being partly involved in trying to articulate what the good life is, 'what it is good to be' (p.5). A vision of the overall good was as important as any method for determining what might be right in any situation, and this requires not just reason but imagination. Hence, metaphysics was not something that required empirical verification as such, but rather provided fuel for the imagination. An example of such a vision might be, for instance, the essential dignity of the human being. Her second key point was the importance of 'consciousness', moral awareness, and that this was 'the fundamental mode or form of moral being' (Murdoch 1993, p.171). Ethics, then, is not about discrete dilemmas or puzzles, which require means (essentially reasoning) to solve. Rather, it involves personal commitment to a vision and response. Hence, for her the stress is on agency and responsibility, and the articulation of that through language. This contrasts with the philosophies that see ethics as being part of a language game. For Murdoch we are the ones who creatively use language (1993). All this puts value before action and even reasoning.

Alasdair McIntyre (1981) builds on such ideas of identity and makes a powerful case for rehabilitating the Aristotelian perspective. He suggests that moral meaning was originally earthed in the context of the religious framework. This has been lost and philosophy *per se* has not filled the gap. The choice, then, is between Aristotle and Nietzsche. Aristotle locates ethics in an intelligible framework that makes sense of moral discourse. Nietzsche suggests that the old moral terminology no longer binds us – indeed, because it robbed us of the freedom to determine our own values, should no longer bind us. McIntyre chooses Aristotle, arguing that ethical meaning is situated in a community of practice, and is communicated not through theory and concepts but rather through stories (and, I would add, all explicit and implicit expressions) that sum up the key virtues of the community. Virtues are at the heart of ethical meaning. In Aristotelian terms, virtues are dispositions to action that occupy the mean not the extreme. Courage, for instance, is neither cowardice nor foolhardiness. Much of this comes down to the virtue of practical wisdom, being able to work through an ethical response that is not about a slavish response to rules.

Underlying the virtues is the *telos* – the Greek word for purpose. This may be the specific purpose of humanity as such, (the ultimate goals of mankind: well-being or happiness, being favourite notions) or the purpose of a person in society. In all this the emphasis is on getting the character right, and good ethical practice following from this. Virtues have, of course, been taken up by many outside philosophies including the so-called 'positive psychology movement', of Seligman and Miller (Miller 2003). One of their favourites is what they see as the virtue of mindfulness – focusing the person, and thus enabling awareness of the self and others. Such awareness forms an excellent basis for prudential ethics.

Charles Taylor builds on the ideas of Murdoch and the neo-Aristotelians. Taylor places moral evaluation at the centre of human identity. Persons understand their identity in large measure by the 'strong evaluations they assert about what is good' (Taylor 1983, p.54). This understanding, in turn, directs their lives. Taylor stresses the direct connection between morality and identity, between value and self-value/esteem. The self involves self-interpretation, and dialogue: 'My discovering of my identity does not mean that I work it out in isolation, but that I negotiate it through dialogue, partly overt, partly internal, with others… My own identity crucially depends upon my dialogical relations with others' (p.67).

Like the neo-Aristotelians, Taylor sees purpose as essential to the self. This is tied, in turn, to responsibility and accountability, which are also essential to the self. If one has purpose and a goal then one is responsible for that. What also emerges from Taylor is an acknowledgement of the importance of community and tradition, an understanding of plurality in community (the many different voices or perspectives within any community), and the importance of dialogic development of identity in that context. Hence, he speaks of the 'plural self' (the many different perspectives on value found within the self) (1983, p.38).

Ricoeur (1992) is a philosopher who comes from a more explicitly religious angle, picking up the themes of narrative, dialogue, identity, and hermeneutics (interpretation). He suggests that it is important to have a transcendent ethical perspective that provides a radical critique of our limited and partial ethical perspectives. In one sense, this is a philosophical reforming of the idea of original sin and teeters close to a moral argument for the existence of God; however, it need not necessarily be seen in theistic terms. It really is about having an unconditional base to ethics, expressed in terms of love. This provides the impetus for creative response. Being unconditional, this cannot find ultimate expression in any community, but we can work towards it and this demands corporate creativity. Importantly, once again Ricoeur's view takes us away from the hands-off approach of philosophy to involvement in that creation. It also focuses on the central role of other virtues, described as theological, faith, hope and love.

The dialogue at the heart of Taylor's views and care in Ricoeur's position are taken up in different ways by other philosophers. Habermas looks to the development of rules of moral discourse through dialogue, such that underlying morality can be discovered (Habermas 1992). Feminist philosophers pick up the importance of an unconditional base to ethics, looking to develop meaning around empathy, trust and care (Koehn 1998).

Each of these is moving into territory that is often seen in terms of spirituality. Taylor explicitly accepts that strong evaluations at the base of decision-making are aligned to spirituality, but finds the term vague (1989). Virtue theory argues that the virtues are embodied in the community stories. Any stories that are told in community will have a ritual context, in which the story can be shared publicly, in education and in community events. This will, in turn, demand that there be story-tellers who are given the responsibility for telling and passing on the meaning of the stories. These will then embody the community identity.

However, whilst these philosophers provide an excellent argument for the connection of ethics with underlying meaning and its continuous development, they do not all come to terms with some of the critical underlying issues, including:

- how community stories can find meaning for the individual without in some sense denying the individual's autonomy

- how any community can handle internal plurality both of stories and interpretation of stories

- how the community can relate to external plurality, without losing its distinctiveness

- how the particular community ethic can relate to a wider view of justice.

Theology

Alongside the philosophers, theologians have further argued the connection of ethics to spirituality in terms of religion. Gamwell (2005) views religion as 'an account of a comprehensive good' (p.114). Such a comprehensive good is represented in 'concepts and symbols, including ritual practices'. Cho (2005) goes further, suggesting that ritual 'performances' are about 'making meaning and identity in everyday life'. 'Action', he argues, ' is the primary context in which moral consciousness and experience materialize'(p.92).

Perhaps the most formidable example of focusing ethics in the ritual of the community is Stanley Hauerwas (Hauerwas and Wells 2004). Hauerwas develops the McIntyre position by arguing that the Christian is schooled in a narrative that teaches him or her how to see the world truthfully. Above all this means seeing what the implications of the narrative are for developing virtues. The narratives that he refers to are to be found at the heart of the Christian rituals, and he is able to suggest that ritual (and therefore Christian worship) is actually the ground of Christian ethical development. Ethics emerges from worship, both in terms of the discovery of meaning and the ethical formation of the person. Hauerwas and Wells (2004) put it this way:

> The liturgy offers ethics a series of ordered practices that shape the character and assumptions of Christians, and suggest habits and models that inform every aspect of the corporate life – meeting people, acknowledging fault and failure, celebrating, thanking, reading, speaking with authority, reflecting on wisdom, naming truth, registering need, bringing about reconciliation, sharing food, renewing purpose. (p.7)

Ethics is thus narrative-dependent, and in order to understand the Christian ethic we have to enter that community. There is thus no universal application of this view of ethics without accepting the Christian faith.

Whilst this approach very firmly reconnects ritual with practice there are still problems associated with it. First, Hauerwas does not recognize the degree of plurality within the Christian Church. Any Christian community is pluri-vocal, as Meeks (1993) notes of the second century church, and tends to develop radical questioning of practice, often informed by those on the margins of the community. Second, Hauerwas does not begin to work through the importance of dialogue and mutual testing, both affective and cognitive, in the development of moral meaning.

Third, like McIntyre, Hauerwas offers no account of personal autonomy in the light of the community narrative. Van der Ven (1996) suggests that narrative is much more complex, involving a dialogue that is critical to the development of the person. The person is both speaker and listener, and writer and reader, and is thus discovering new aspects of self with each articulation in context. These new aspects are, in turn, open to critique of the self and others. What is true of the person is also true of the learning community.

Fourth, because ethics is focused around the shaping experience of the liturgy there is no way in which Hauerwas' view of ethics can begin to dialogue with others outside the church. He admits that the church does not always get things right, but argues that this has to be sorted out within the community, because critiques from outside have no relevance. In short, the Hauerwas position makes ethics relative and dependent upon the particular community. This then means that it is difficult to have any sense of dialogue with other communities, without accepting the underlying belief system of the other community.

Religious ethics

Developments in religious ethics have, in the past decade, begun to point to ways in which the tension between community meaning and moral and personal autonomy can be addressed. First, there has been significant critique of dependency upon moral theories. A good example of this is utilitarianism, which argues that the basis of ethics is maximizing the good for the greatest number. The much-cited problem with this is that it does not offer any view of what the good is. Without that, this so-called ethical theory has little meaning, and, indeed, is shown up for what it is – a calculus, a method for calculating what might be a right response.

As Lovin (2005) puts it 'moral theories are, at best, accounts of the central convictions that shape a particular way of life' (p.25). Attempts to build a general theory unrelated to any particular way of life tend to distort the moral meaning. An attempt to argue for one moral theory also runs the danger of imposing a particular, usually Western, view of ethics on different cultures (Lovin 2005). Lovin concludes that moral theories can be useful without being the ground of ethics, just as cultural foundations of ethics are important but cannot be accepted uncritically.

Second, Fasching and Dechant (2001) develop this point about critical challenge, and suggest that religious scriptures have a tradition of 'audacious challenge', alongside any stress on obedience (p.172). They focus on the Jewish tradition of audacity, set down in the sacred stories and which models figures contending with God. A good example is Abraham, involved in arguing with God about how His action against Sodom will kill the 'righteous with the wicked' (Genesis 18:23).

As Meeks (1993) notes, the early Christian church developed through argument and debate. It is precisely through these arguments that the church develops its moral character. This same tradition is seen throughout the church history. Luther, for instance, fights for the freedom of the individual to relate directly to God and not through the church/priesthood. St Francis wrestles with the power and authority of the Christian church. Fasching and Dechant note the most recent challenge to orthodox thinking and practice from feminist theologians.

Fasching and Dechant suggest that audacious challenge is more than a means to the end of moral awareness. It involves a wrestling that is in itself a core process in the development of moral awareness. They note similar traditions of challenge in Buddhist, Hindu and Islamic communities.

This suggests that there is a robust tradition in which ethics (as working out what justice or goodness means) can contend with God or the view of the Church. Indeed, it suggests that such a view is important in the development of any ethical meaning. It points to a view of the relationship between ethics and spirituality that involves interaction and mutual challenge, rather than simply ethical decision-making arising from an unquestioned spiritual ground.

This begins to address the core issue of how spirituality, in whatever form, relates to autonomy, and suggests that Plato's dilemma (see p.17) is false. We can only begin to ascertain what God wants through sustained wrestling with the traditions and communities of religion and community. I will suggest in subsequent chapters that such a challenge can come from both within and outside any formal religion. This also offers a way through a second issue, highlighted by Grelle (2005), that of plurality.

Grelle suggests that the very different views of religious ethics have to be respected and can only be understood in dialogue and in context. Respecting such plurality and developing dialogue around it can lead not just to some shared anodyne principles or values, but also to shared commitment to practice in context. It is in that focus on practice, I would suggest, lies the real possibility of discovering universal values that are meaningful. Hence, Gaita (2000) can argue that the universal can only be known in the particular. Spohn (1997) also argues that spirituality and ethics come together in practice, not least through communities of practice and the related virtues.

Not all religious writers go down the line of plurality, or of dialogue. Holloway (1999) and Milbank (1990) represent two other views, at different extremes. Holloway argues against those who would say that it is only in the spirituality of this or that religion that one can begin to find an adequate basis for ethics. He rehearses the historical arguments about formal religion's abuse of power. Holloway suggests that Christian morality has often been used to prevent genuine moral reflection amongst Christians. He urges us to pursue a morality that is based in moral reasoning, and does not use God to convince. The problem about Holloway's position is that he does not give full weight to the importance of engaging spiritual meaning, including working it out at an affective level and as part of one's moral identity – as part of moral reasoning. Hence, he runs the danger of throwing the baby out with the bath-water.

Milbank, on the other hand, argues that it is only possible to convince through the God narrative. Put briefly, he argues all postmodern secular thinkers are essentially negative, influenced in this by Nietzsche and Descartes. The negativity is shown in the postmodern stress on nihilism, which leads, in turn, to violence. In contrast to this secular perspective, Milbank notes the Christian meta-narrative. This stands out as being distinctively worked around peace, together with a view of gift and reciprocity focused in narrative. Hence, he argues that the task of the Christian church is not to enter into dialogue, but to 'out narrate' the other views, so that this essentially truthful view held by the church triumphs.

There is not space here to do Milbank's view full justice. However, I feel it important to raise several problems it presents. First, he does not grasp the pluralistic nature of communities, and thus polarizes the debate. I would point only to how some, including Pope Benedict (in his 2006 Regensburg lecture) view the Muslim faith as a community of violence (Schall 2007). They clearly fail to take into account different Muslim subgroups who are devoutly pacifist. In fact, one with a very large following in Turkey, the Nursi Muslims, has a theology of peace that is close to that of Pope John Paul II (Michel 2005). Second, Milbank posits a negative view of all postmodern thinkers that has little foundation (Hart 2004, Reader 1997). Third, he assumes a univocal view of the Christian faith that has never actually existed. Historically, a peace-centred church has only been a recent phenomenon. Finally, he fails to grasp the nature of narrative. The very idea of 'out-narrating' the other narratives ignores the reflective and learning function and nature of narrative. Later I go on to argue that narrative is the vehicle of spirituality and that it provides a means not simply to state a position but also to critique and develop one's own tradition. Furthermore, Milbank's approach ignores the possibility that there could, in other narratives, be things that the Christian narrative might learn from or relate to.

In Milbank's approach it is difficult to see how there can be any dialogue between Christian spirituality and the ethical world beyond.

Moral development

The disciplines of moral development and character education have also been involved in similar issues about determining ethics. Lapsley and Navarez (2006) note how work on character education has involved giving attention to pedagogy that can develop virtues. The transmission model of pedagogy mirrors the view of a community transmitting or modelling core virtues; the democratic models of pedagogy look to develop virtues through dialogue. Mustakova-Possardt (2004) suggests the importance of the development of critical moral consciousness, and argues that spirituality is a critical part of that. Such a consciousness involves not simply an awareness of the other, and their values and beliefs, but of the self and the ground of one's own world view and values. Such a view moves away from what she refers to as 'soft relativism' (the simple acceptance of every different view and the impossibility of a universal perspective) (p.248), and thus revisits Taylor's ideas about the plural self. I will return to this and the work of Fasching and Dechant in Chapter 3.

Summing up

In conclusion, I would argue that there now seems to be an increasing concern to link spirituality with ethics in such a way that ethics are not dependent upon a particular view of spirituality, and which affirms both individual autonomy and community without slipping into meaningless relativism. This concern is magnified in health and social care, where the autonomy of the patient or client is very much the cornerstone of any professional ethic. We may disagree about just what someone's autonomy might mean, but recognize that some sense of both freedom to make decisions and responsibility for those decisions is central to it (Kendrick and Robinson, 2002). If that is to be respected then it follows that spirituality has at the least to be seen as part of any view of autonomy. Indeed, spirituality that involves a conscious reflection on underlying significant meaning can be seen to strengthen autonomy and responsibility, as Taylor (1989, p.14) implies in his idea of 'strong evaluation'. This, however, demands a view of spirituality that is clear and inclusive, with the stress being on how the person can reflect on and develop their belief and value system in relation to their communities. Equally important is that this should be straightforward, and can easily be addressed in practice. A common approach to this will enable better team working that can fully address the issues that may arise for any patient or client.

The way forward would seem to be to explore the idea of a broader spirituality – one that includes religion – in the context of a critical moral consciousness. In Chapter 2 I go on to outline such a spirituality, one that can enable engagement and reflection from anyone and which could be enabled by different care professions. Then in Chapter 3 I will show how this can provide a framework for ethical reflection that takes underlying beliefs seriously.

2

Exploring Spirituality

Case Study

Enid moves into the hospital ward. She has been suffering pain for some time from her hip and is about to have an operation. Prior to the operation she seems to be distressed. A nurse sits down with her and asks her how she is feeling. Enid says, 'I feel so down. I have been looking forward to getting this hip sorted. But now I feel frightened and depressed. The more I feel frightened and depressed, the more I feel ashamed.'

The nurse encourages Enid to reflect on these feeling and see what is involved.

'I feel ashamed because I know that God is with me and I realize that this is the right thing to do, but I feel frightened. I feel that my faith is weak, I am not trusting God enough to let go, and be healed by this operation.'

'That is OK,' replies the nurse, 'just because you feel frightened before an op doesn't mean that you have lost your faith, or you are letting God down. I would think he would understand what you are feeling and want to care for you, wouldn't he. Why don't you send for your pastor or someone in the church. We can call them for you.'

Enid becomes very agitated at this point, verging on tears, 'No please, you mustn't. The pastor is a good man but he will just tell me to trust in God, and I know I should, but I really am finding that difficult. In any case it's not just what will happen in the operation that scares me, it's what will happen afterwards.

Whilst I've had this hip I've started to think. Sometimes it has been great. For the first time in 15 years of a family people have done things for me, and I have not felt guilty about it. But I've pushed myself as well and worked through the pain 'cos that's what I'm about, being a good mother and a wife. That's what the Bible tells us and I believe it. But just lately I've begun to think, is it worth it? Is it worth the pain? Do I really want to just get patched up so that I can get back to doing what other people want. And the more that I think that, the more ashamed I feel, and the more I feel I am losing my spirit.'

At this point she holds her hand out to the nurse. 'You remind me of my granddaughter,' she said. 'Could you sit with me for a bit.'

Introduction

Whatever was happening to Enid here it's clear that it mattered a great deal to her. Two of the most important things in her life were being questioned and such that she felt she was losing what she referred to as her 'spirit'. Clearly, there are many different views as to what the spirit might be. These include:

- a transcendental or essential dimension of life (Highfield 1992; Reed 1987)

- a force or energy (Boyd 1995; King and Dein 1998; Sims 1994), and

- life-meaning and purpose (Doyle 1992; Hiatt 1986; Joseph 1998).

However, rather than each of these representing distinct models, these can be taken together to indicate important aspects of the human spirit that were all central in Enid's crisis. In this chapter I will therefore begin by looking in more detail at the meaning of the spirit and spirituality and then go on to develop a three-fold definition of spirituality.

The experience of transition

It is commonplace to say that explicit reflection on spirituality often emerges during crisis, and therefore is to be expected in the experience of illness. However, as Bridges (1980) notes, times of transition are a normal part of growth and development for all persons and groups, and not just in times of medical crisis. Bridges suggests four characteristics of the experience of transition – characteristics that lie at the root of much that has been described in the literature as spiritual pain or distress:

- *Disengagement.* This involves a breakdown of relationships and shared meaning that helped constitute a sense of the self.

- *Disidentification.* The person tries to rediscover her identity in old patterns of faith but cannot identify with them.

- *Disenchantment.* This involves a loss of faith in old perceptions of reality. This often brings with it feelings of anger, resentment, grief, loss, guilt, and confusion. It can also bring with it a sense of liberation and new possibilities.

- *Disorientation.* This is the cumulative effect of the previous three experiences and involves a loss of direction, energy and motivation, and much time and energy being put into trying to grasp meaning in any of this.

Enid was experiencing such a crisis; and it was all the more a crisis for her because she had rarely before, if ever, reflected on, or had to test her purpose and meaning in life.

What is 'spirit'?

The word spirit comes from the Latin *spiritus* (Hebrew *ruach*, Greek *pneuma*), meaning breath, wind, and even life principle. It is that which is vital to and animates the self. As such the spirit is not primarily about ideas but is about lived experience, something that brings together values, feelings and thoughts. Hence, the spirit is evidenced not so much in doctrines but in action and attitude – through being embodied. Doctrines that assist understanding of what that spirit is can be developed – not least to help maintain that spirit – but these are not the spirit as such. This view of the spirit has a strong sense of holism – involving the integration of affective, cognitive and physical elements, and making it impossible to isolate the spiritual from the physical. The spirit, then, is a dynamic reality that expresses itself in the body. This can apply also to groups. Hence, it is possible to speak of 'team spirit' or 'company spirit', revealed in the way that members of the team are integrated and work together to express purpose and achieve tasks.

A holistic view of the spirit is well supported by empirical evidence that charts the relationship between feelings, thoughts, the body and the social and physical environment (Swinton 2001). Importantly, the word 'spirit' here refers to the sense of life (that which animates), the identity (that which particularly characterizes the person or group), and the qualities of that person or group. Enid specifically felt that she had lost her animating purpose and identity and, with that, her usual resilience and hope.

This holistic view of the spirit contrasts sharply with the more dualistic view of the spirit as something separate from the body. This idea arose from the philosophy of Plato and ultimately led to the view that the 'spirit' was that which was incorruptible, (hence immortal, and of the highest value) and the body was that which was corrupting and corruptible, and of the least value (Edwards 1999). Whilst such dualism has been very influential and continues in many popular ways of thinking it has little in empirical terms to support it. Moreover, it tends to lead to a fragmentation of human experience.

For Enid, the spirit had also involved something beyond the self. It was difficult for her to hold onto her spirit without reaching out beyond the self and being aware of the *other* – whether that was another person, including all her family and faith community, or God's presence mediated by another person. Some writers on the spirit have tried to locate it purely in the transcendent, that which is beyond the self. However, clearly for Enid it is precisely this that she is questioning. An awareness of the other was critical to awareness of her spirit as she experienced the fear that threatened to overwhelm her sense of self. This suggests an interactive relationship between the self and the other, out of which emerges the spirit and an awareness of the spirit. Reed (1998) tries to focus on this relationship by distinguishing between the soul (the holistic essence of the person) and the spirit, that which is beyond the person and which the person responds to. It is in openness to the other, and in dialogue with the other, that the person develops awareness of her essential self. On the grounds that attempting to distinguish between the soul and spirit can be confusing, I prefer to talk in terms of the spirit as the holistic and experiential essence of the self that is discovered in and through relating to the 'other'. For Enid this was explored with the nurse precisely because she reminded her of her granddaughter. It emerged that her granddaughter represented a route into her church and family that was neither demanding nor judgemental. It later became clear that Enid could be her childlike and vulnerable self with her granddaughter and still feel part of the family and church, while the pastor represented the demands of the church, the rest of her family made her feel guilty for being in hospital. After spending a quarter of an hour chatting about this with the nurse, Enid began to feel more centred.

Many writers have suggested that the spirit can be regarded as a power or force that is at the heart of personal growth, allowing the person to transcend the self and thus learn, and in some way integrate, personal experience (Goddard 1995). Enid began to develop power once she felt able to let go and to relate to the two core groups in her life as someone in need. However, such power was something that emerged *from* the relationships as she gradually became more aware of them. Understanding these relationships better enabled her to be more aware of her essential self, thus reducing anxiety and increasing her sense of well-being, and thus empowering her. Although Enid still experienced real ambivalence about her role and expectations in the church and family, she began at least to see what she could receive from (as well as give to) her spiritual homes.

Swinton (2001) argues that in such contexts the concept of power or energy is used in a metaphorical way. To speak of the spirit as like a force or involving a force, is quite different from the idea of the spirit as energy itself.

The spirit can also be strongly connected to the development of significant meaning. Ellison (1983) describes the connection in this way:

It is the *spirit* of human beings which enables and motivates us to search for meaning and purpose in life, to seek the supernatural or some meaning which transcends us, to wonder about our origins and our identities, to require morality and equity. (p.331)

In another sense it might be said that the spirit itself is discovered in and through the struggle with meaning in practice. For Enid this meant a difficult period of reflection, trying to locate her spirit in the midst of her fear and confusion, and that reflection was destined to continue throughout her treatment and recovery. As Enid later reflected on her experience she was able to develop a stronger sense of her spirit, but one that was complex and involved very different needs and sometimes conflicting values. For Enid this meant a very different approach, demanding regular reflection.

What is spirituality?

Spirituality is about the practice and outworking of the spirit and the ways in which someone connects its different aspects and relationships and sustains and understands it. As we will see, this can involve the spirituality of any particular individual or that which is developed in and through the disciplines and practices of a group. It is often a combination of both. Essentially, then, spirituality is relation and action centred, and about making connections between one's spirit and these different aspects of life.

It is also possible to refer to spirituality as an academic discipline, involving systematic research that reflects upon such practice and the meanings that may emerge from that. Spirituality, however, cannot be simply an academic discipline, precisely because the reflection it involves is holistic and embodied, requiring more than just intellectual understanding and awareness.

A working definition of spirituality can involve three parts (Robinson, Kendrick and Brown 2003), as summed up in Box 2.1.

- Developing *awareness* and *appreciation* of the other (including the self, the other person, the group, the environment and, where applicable, deity).
- Developing the capacity to respond to the other. This involves putting spirituality into practice, *embodying* spirituality, and thus the continued relationship with the other.
- Developing *ultimate life meaning* based upon awareness and appreciation of, and response to, the other.

Box 2.1 A working definition of spirituality from Robinson, Kendrick and Brown (2003)

I will now go on to to examine each part of this definition in more detail.

Awareness and appreciation of the other

By 'the other' here I mean the self, another person, a larger group, the environment and the divine.

THE SELF

Ricoeur (1992) argues that it is reasonable to speak of the self as other because in one sense the self is, indeed, simply one amongst others and so is an other to someone else. In another sense we can speak of a person moving beyond the self – the psychological distance achieved enables the person to begin to see her self as other. Hence, we can speak of self-transcendence. This self-transcendence enables, first, some increased awareness of oneself as a whole person, with a wide range of thoughts, feelings, physical experience, practice, and relationships. For Enid this was not easy. She only began to achieve this transcendence through articulating the contrasting and seemingly conflicting concerns around her family and church, as well as her physical pain and weakness and her affective pain manifested in fear and loneliness. Such transcendence didn't magically take away the pain and fear that threatened to engulf her but it did allow her to begin to rise above and reflect on those feelings and perceptions and to work through what they involved. As van der Ven (1996) comments, 'Awareness of the self leads to the capacity to develop dialogue with the self, something which distinguishes human experience from other species' (p.108).

Second, there can be an awareness of the self as being both same and different. Difference is about the uniqueness of each person, and is essential for the particular identity of the self. However, the self cannot be understood if it is completely different from others. Indeed, complete difference makes someone into a stranger, someone whom one cannot identify with. Equally, if the self is simply the same as others, located purely as one of many, with no distance from the group, there is the danger of a loss of identity. Enid was locked into both of these aspects. She felt alienated from the two major communities that gave her life meaning. She thought of herself as unable to accept their demands and saw herself as being strange and different from them. Her granddaughter, and the nurse, however, represented a comforting accepting presence, very much the same as her. She became aware that the self is revealed as essentially ambiguous – the same as others but different. To work through the issues she had to accept that she was both different from some people and the same as others.

Third, awareness of the self involves awareness of the limitations of the self. Holistic awareness of the different aspects of the self can thus never lead to or point to wholeness, in the sense of completeness. For Enid, the key limitation was her inability to fulfil the demands of others, and behind that was an awareness of her mortality. As she focused on that she was increasingly aware that she was interdependent not independent. In practice this inevitably means acceptance, in certain contexts, of dependence without any sense of shame, which was in this case beautifully summed up in the sight of Enid holding her hand out to the nurse. She reached an appreciation of the self, as both limited but also creative, as interdependent but also dependent.

Finally, the self is an embodied (somatic) being, as well as one of emotion and intellect. This somatic awareness includes an awareness of one's sexuality – one's sexual identity and being. This area is a good example of the way in which historically there has been a fragmentation of the person. The spirit was often seen as not just simply distinct from the body but also antipathetic to it and thus to sexuality. Sexuality is by definition ambiguous, both a wonderful experience and expression of the embodied person and also something fraught with risk and moral challenge. The easiest way to handle this culturally was often to simply separate the spirit (good) from the sexual (bad). As Avis (1989) notes, the result was to devalue the physical and sexual and thus to retreat from real awareness of the self and other, in all its ambiguity and risk. Spirituality, rather, involves the integration of sexuality with the self and looks to find meaning in relationships that include this (Helminiak 1998).

INTERPERSONAL RELATIONSHIPS

Awareness of another person, like awareness of the self, involves recognition of difference and sameness. For the other to be simply different means that there is no point of common humanity through which one can relate to them. Hence, the person who is seen purely as different is often literally dehumanized, seen as enemy as well as stranger. This is the spiritual dynamic at the heart of racism, expressed ultimately in the Holocaust (Bauman 1989).

Equally, to see the other as purely the same can lead to a loss of identity, that which makes the other unique. As Kahlil Gibran (1995) notes that marriage requires some distance and space between the two:

Fill each other's cup but drink not from one cup.

Give one another of your bread but eat not from the same loaf.

> Sing and dance together and be joyous, but let each one of you be alone, even as the strings of a lute are alone though they quiver with the same music. (p.5)

The sameness that is recognized in the other provides the basis for trust and collaboration – it enables the person to see the other. But the difference provides the basis for continued learning, disclosure, and discovery. The personal and interpersonal are then connected in the self. It is not possible to be aware of the holistic and distinctive nature of the self without developing awareness of the other. Equally, it is not possible to see the other without seeing something of the self in the other (Buber 1937).

THE LARGER GROUP

Beyond one-to-one relationships is corporate or cultural spirituality. For Enid the corporate identity of the family and the church had provided her with both a sense of belonging and security, and also a sense of active participation and contribution. Once more this provides the dimensions of sameness and difference. Such a dimension is part of what it means to be human, as Mbiti (1990) writes in the context of African spirituality:

> A person cannot detach himself from the religion of his group, for to do so is to be severed from his roots, his foundation, his context of security, his kinship and the entire group of those who make him aware of his own existence. (Mbiti 1990, p.2)

This element in society is increasingly being lost under the stress of consumerism and individualism, which tend to stress the contract nature of groups, i.e. groups formed from individual choice and with no historical or moral claim on the person outside of a mutually agreed contract. Groups, as a result, can easily become instrumental – simply used by the person for his or her own ends.

Increased awareness of any group reveals its complexity and ambiguity. Every group, for instance, has both community elements (ways in which the members relate to and support each other), and institutional elements (ways in which the group manages, orders and maintains itself). The institutional element is often seen as the enemy of community, with bureaucracy replacing relationships, creating distance between individuals or subgroups, or defending the group from the outside. Nonetheless, the institution aspect is necessary for the continued running of the group.

Each group will have narratives that try to articulate the purpose and values of the groups, and rules and regulations for the maintenance of order. Each group, in different ways, takes on a life or character of its own, expressed through narrative and practice. Each group will also have very different sub-groups that relate in different ways to the whole group. The group will also relate in different ways beyond itself, possibly even having a purpose that is greater than it own particular good or the good of its members. Hence, the spirituality of the group involves plurality.

On reflection Enid also recognized that she was part of, and had faith in, several groups. Multiple group membership might be thought to militate against the corporate spirituality of Mbiti. However, in fact we are all inevitably members of more than one group throughout our lives including our:

- given family
- chosen family, developed through partnerships entered into
- school and institutions of higher or further education
- local community
- work
- interest groups
- culture groups
- faith groups.

One group may be more central to someone than others, with the person placing more faith in it, yet all are part of the framework or meaning structure of the person. Moreover, being a member of more than one group can help to clarify both the wider meaning of a group or groups, and the identity of the person. Johannes van der Ven refers to 'intertextuality', the dialogue that the self develops with the narratives or texts of all the different groups and through which personal moral and spiritual meaning is developed (van der Ven 1996, p.258). In other words, there is rarely simply one narrative alone that provides someone's life-meaning. Life-meaning arises out of the different narratives in dialogue. This is stressed in the work of Kelly (1990) who reflects not simply on the spirituality centred round different groups but also on that of a nation itself – in his case Australia.

THE ENVIRONMENT

The term 'transcendent' can be applied to all of the categories considered so far. However, it is most often used with the last two categories we will consider – those of the wider environment and the divine. The word 'environment' can be used to describe anything from the physical and social environment that surrounds us, to the environment that is created through art, to nature itself. The natural environment, of course, can be so vast that the sense of otherness it creates is overwhelming. Standing at the foot of the Bridal Veil Falls at Niagara, for instance, it is difficult not to feel a part of some greater whole, through a literally breathtaking experience, which can lead to a momentary loss of the sense of the self as something separate. However, just as there are physical boundaries at Niagara for safety, psychological boundaries are necessary between people as without a knowledge of the self over against the other, there could be no actual conscious awareness of the other.

Awareness of the environment as another presence is not simply about recognizing difference. The spirituality of the Lakota Native Americans, for instance, perceives the environment in terms of its own familiar social networks of belonging. Hence, a Lakotan will pray, 'for all my relatives', including, animals, birds, plants, water, rocks and so on (Lartey 1997, p.121). In the same way St Francis of Assisi was able to refer to 'dear mother earth' or 'brother sun and sister moon'.

A genuine awareness of the environment reveals ambiguities and complexities in one's relationship with it. Humans depend upon the environment for sustenance, and it depends upon mankind, for protection and responsible stewardship. At the heart of this is an interconnectedness that sees humans as not existing as separate from the environment, but as affecting it by whatever they do (McFague 1997). The environment is also a place of risk. Weather can change in a short time and if care is not taken can easily lead to injury or death. The animal world is not the same as the human world and, if not respected, can also lead to death. Hence, Otto (1923) pinpoints the human's ambivalent response to the environment as a mixture of fascination and fear.

THE DIVINE

For many, the divine epitomizes the transcendent. Any deity tends to be seen as being totally other – as all-powerful, perfect, and so on. This sense of otherness informs common views of the concepts of the holy or sacred, meaning 'set apart'. For Enid, however, the critical point about her faith object, the ground of her being, was that she be able to relate to God directly. She could not begin to understand Him or be aware of Him as simply the transcendent being. Indeed, by definition such a being is alien, and cannot be understood. Characteristically the more that the otherness of the divine is stressed the more he or she is seen as a figure to be feared, and thus to be placated with sacrifices and the like. It is critical then to see the sameness in any divinity as well as the difference. This is expressed well in the Hebrew *imago deo* doctrine – that man was made in the image of God (Genesis 5:1). It is also expressed in Christian spirituality through the idea of God becoming man in the form of Jesus Christ. The human face of God is what changed the relationship from a tyrannical God who is to be feared, to one who identifies with His people. It is precisely that imminence that Enid needed at her bedside, and which could only be communicated through the presence of an other.

There are, of course, many different expressions of the spirituality of the divine, but all seek some sense of the divine in the present 'known' experience, and all have some sense of the complexity of the divine. Ascribing human qualities to the divine has, of course, been common in many religions, from Ancient Greece to Hinduism.

SUMMING UP SO FAR

Even at this stage it is clear that the positive spirituality being argued for in this book is essentially relational and reflective. It cannot be static, or simply be a set of meanings forced upon experience. Moreover, it is well suited to the idea of a postmodern time, precisely because it recognizes that anyone's spirituality may involve relationships with many different groups. Hence, by its very nature, spirituality is not likely to depend on a meta-narrative, one story that gives meaning to experience.

In slightly different ways awareness of self and others involves knowledge of:

- the holistic other, involving cognitive, affective and somatic elements and as connected to and affecting a network of others

- the other as both same and different, and hence ambiguous

- the interdependence of different others

- the nature of the other as always emerging, as always learning and therefore never totally knowable

- the other as involving both imminence (awareness of the self) and transcendence (a movement beyond the self).

The second element of the definition of spirituality is that of developing the capacity to respond to the other.

The capacity to respond

I would argue that response to the other is essentially about the articulation of spirituality in practice. It involves roles that express something of one's relationship to others, and one's contribution towards these relationships. The response to the other can be seen in terms of *vocation* (calling), or response to the calling, or needs, of the other and in terms of placing *faith* in the other. The idea of vocation has tended to be either restricted to a particular purpose or profession or, in practice to the Christian spirituality, with God calling the Christian. However, in terms of a broader human spirituality all the different others 'call' the person in some way:

- The environment calls the person or group to be aware of the complexities and interconnectedness and to respond with responsible stewardship.

- The group calls the person or other groups to be aware and to respond to need with a particular contribution.

- The other person calls for response as his or her needs are disclosed.

McFadyen (1990) argues that such a call is the basis of personal identity. Any calling, of course, has to be tested, and as discussed below, also involves negotiation about how responsibility is to be shared.

The response to the other may be one of accepting need *for* the other in some way. We need the environment and community for our continued existence and different groups for our social and physical well-being. Acknowledging that need, and the way in which the other fulfils it, enables us to begin put faith in other. This is, in itself, a response to that person, group or environment.

The response of one person to the other then becomes an embodiment of spirituality, life-meaning in action. In this sense, the response is another aspect of transcendence, with action going beyond the self. The embodiment may be individual or collaborative. Importantly, the embodiment of this spirituality is in itself a working out of the life-meaning, not simply the applying of a set meaning to the situation. Indeed, it is not possible to fully understand any life-meaning other than in and through the practical testing and outworking of it (Ricoeur 1992).

Developing life-meaning

Life-meaning can be seen in two broad ways, doctrinal and existential. First, there are doctrines or philosophies that attempt to encapsulate something about the nature of life, including the social and physical environment. These form the basis of our belief about how the world is and how we might best operate within that world. Scientific doctrines provide a clear view of the limitations and possibilities of our human context. Philosophical and theological doctrines, in contrast, provide the basis of how we might make sense of that world and so respond to it. Hence, ancient religious doctrines, for instance, set out how God related to the world and therefore how we might respond to it. However, life-meaning in the light of the holistic and community perspective cannot be simply confined to conceptual beliefs. It is also located in and understood in two broader ways:

- *Holistic meaning.* This involves existential whole-person awareness.

- *Value-based meaning.* Meaning here is discovered in the value the person recognizes in herself and others. Such value may be based on a sense of unconditional acceptance from the other and a sense of worth, and any contribution to the other and the wider community, a sense of purpose.

HOLISTIC MEANING

In my view, knowledge and awareness involves four levels of meaning:

- cognitive (to do with ideas about the world)

- affective (to do with emotions)

- somatic (to do with 'body language', including tactile communication), and

- interpersonal.

All four can involve awareness of all of these aspects in the other and how these affect each other. Once again, this cannot be a complete awareness. In most situations that challenge the individual that person reflects and discovers different aspects of the self that may have been previously unrecognized or not accepted. Such awareness is mediated through one or more of the routes of knowledge. In Enid's case the somatic knowledge (provided by holding the nurse's hand) was able to mediate the interpersonal knowledge (about the nurse and her granddaughter) and affective knowledge about the nature of care from both people – all of which gave her a sense of security. Later conflicting cognitive meaning was worked through as she articulated her story to the nurse and eventually to her pastor, enabling feelings and beliefs to come together. The experience was not made sense of simply in terms of doctrinal truths but rather in terms of how Enid retained her holistic identity in the light of her intense feelings of fear, loneliness, isolation, anger, and frustration.

MEANING AND VALUE

Trying to make sense of life, especially in a crisis, takes one beyond simply doctrines to questions of purpose and to searching for hope and relationships in which we can put our faith. Locating and developing our faith is therefore a core part of finding spiritual meaning. That spiritual meaning rests on the value that those relationships give one. For some this may be conditional value – 'I am of value if I please the other person/group.' For others it can be unconditional value – 'I am of value without having to fulfil any conditions.' For most people there is something of both in relationships of significance. A person's value is thus central to finding meaning and, as shall be seen later, central to ethical meaning. It is not surprising that in the experience of illness it is often the patient's faith (in ideas, groups or persons) – and with that their underlying sense of value – that is severely challenged.

James Fowler (1990) has developed extensive work on faith, suggesting that there are different kinds of faith, seen as stages. He defines faith in two ways:

(1) the foundational dynamic of trust and loyalty underlying selfhood and relationships. In this sense faith is a human universal, a generic quality of human beings;

(2) a holistic way of knowing, in which persons shape their relationships with the self, others and the world in the light of and apprehension of and by transcendence. (p.394)

Fowler refers to two other views of faith that are specifically religious: the response to the gift of salvation; and obedient assent to revealed truth.

Faith, in its generic sense, is very much belief *in* an other. This is in contrast to belief *that* or belief *about*. It is possible, for instance, to believe in the concept of God, or *that* God exists, without making the belief *in* him the basis of life. Belief in may involve any of the others noted above, or ideas related to them. Clearly such faith will vary from complete trust in the other to partial or working trust. The latter can build faith on the other whilst being aware of its limitations.

Such belief directly affects practice. Fowler argues that faith develops through discernible stages. Each of these stages is about the development of the self and the relationship of the person to the different others.

STAGES OF FAITH

Fowler (1996) proposes seven stages of faith, which he locates at different ages. These are very much based upon the work of Kohlberg (1984), who built Piaget's work in the development of moral meaning and judgement into three phases (each further subdivided into two stages).

Undifferentiated or primal faith (infancy)

This is a pre-linguistic and pre-conceptual stage in which the infant begins to form a disposition towards an environment that is gradually being recognized as distinct from the self. This stage forms the cradle of trust or mistrust and of self worth based on unconditional or conditional grounds.

Intuitive-projective faith (ages 2–6)

This stage builds upon the development of language and the imagination. With no cognitive operations that can test perceptions and thus reverse beliefs, children grasp experience in and through powerful images. The child is thus attentive to ritual and gesture.

Mythic-literal faith (7–12)

This sees a reliance on stories and rules, and the narrative that is implied in the family faith experience. The lived faith of the family – through practice, ritual, and belief – is valued in a concrete and literal sense. This can also involve some testing of the story's meaning.

Synthetic-conventional faith (12–21)

The child in this stage moves on to search for 'a story of my stories'. This involves the development of life-meaning in general and that person's particular life-meaning. At one level this is a product of the development of new cognitive abilities referred to by Piaget (1965) as early formal operations. At the same time the developing life-meaning is built up of the original faith system, and thus compiled of conventional elements. This faith is often accompanied by a strong sense of the need to keep together the faith group as a priority.

Individuative-reflective faith (21–30)

Now, faith meaning is more personally chosen and believed. There is an awareness that one's view is different from others, and can be expressed in abstract terms. The faith developed at this stage is for the sake of the person and for making sense of his or her life in family or community. It is not developed primarily for the unity of the family.

Conjunctive faith (31–40)
In this stage many of the different ideas and perspectives, and the resulting tensions and paradoxes, are worked at. Previously unexamined, these are now held together in balance, with an openness to the perspectives of others. This sees a deepening of appreciation of the complex nature of faith and life-meaning.

Universalising faith (40 and beyond)
This not so much a stage of faith as a category of individuals who have developed a coherent faith that is grounded in the 'other', and which enables them to live unfettered by self-concern. Membership of this group is very rare and includes, for example Mahatma Ghandi and Martin Luther King.

Criticisms of the Fowler stage approach include arguments that it is too cognitive and intellectual and too individualistic. Others argue that the stages are normative, with the later stages being seen as superior to the early ones. Others question the adequacy of the research (Parks 1992). However, such criticisms can be refuted.

First, although Fowler sees the stages (as Kohlberg does), to be invariant, sequential and hierarchical, i.e. they have to be gone through in turn, he does not advocate that they be taken too rigorously. They are a useful tool for noting characteristics of faith development, and which can help the practitioner to be aware of needs. Second, Fowler does argue for a broader, rational view of faith including affective knowledge. The intellectual component of spirituality does not make it a superior form. Third, he argues that the needs expressed in the earlier stages are not left behind. Moreover, as noted above, these spiritual needs may be most apparent in times of crisis or transition. Someone who is bereaved, for instance, may need the safety of a simple child-like faith to carry him or her through the pain, or even to express the pain. Later a more complex view of faith may emerge as the complexity of the bereaved's relationship to the deceased is worked through. Fowler also suggests that the faith of the earlier stages is carried over and reworked into the new faith. Indeed, without this any sense of affective continuity is gone. Enid finally worked through to stage five where she did not have to be dominated by the demands of family and church, but in reaching out and finding faith, albeit temporarily, in the nurse she was acknowledging the need to have a much simpler affective faith in another at that point in her experience.

I would argue that other critical aspects of meaning in spirituality include:

- The development of purpose, in relation to the other.

- The generation of hope. Hope has often been associated with some quasi-mystical concept based upon future promises. Hence, some religious expressions of spirituality see hope as based upon the promise of life after death (Edwards 1999). The problem with this approach is the danger of forming hope around a concept. Although this may satisfy cognitive knowledge it has little to offer affective understanding, not least where the person is suffering pain or anxiety. Enid's anxiety was not going to be dispelled by doctrine. She needed the presence of a person and a sense of her spirit, in relation to others, to find meaning that was relevant to her experience. Enid's hope was based in an other (Robinson 1998).

- Addressing and resolving relational conflicts and problems. This may involve reconciliation and forgiveness. Hence, it is difficult to confine spirituality to the personal realm, since it also affects society and even politics (Selby 1983).

I will examine each of these three meaning dimensions more closely in subsequent chapters.

The development of meaning in spirituality can thus focus on holistic, existential and value meaning, which relates to the different relationships between the self and the other. In particular, it focuses on the development of *faith* in the other, and *hope* – which is generated through significant purpose and function, leading to resolution of conflict and possibly reconciliation and forgiveness.

As discussed earlier, one aspect of spirituality in this is about finding meaning through transcendence. Hence, Reed sums up spirituality as:

> the human propensity to find meaning in and through self-transcendence; it is evident in perspective and behaviours that express a sense of relatedness to a transcendent dimension, or to something greater than the self and may or may not include formal religious practice. (Reed 1998, p.50)

I shall return to this in Chapters 3 and 4.

SPIRITUALITY AND TRAGEDY

Finally, it must be noted that the view of spirituality being developed in this book is not simplistic or unrealistic. It does not suggest that everything can be worked out 'in the end', because at times humans have to make sense of, or live with, complex tragedy. Rather, it is a spirituality that is aware of dangers and risks. Indeed, the very action of reaching out to the other is one of risk, not least because it involves some loss of control. The other also may involve danger, not least in the physical environment. Ironically, that very danger can lead to increased awareness. So one can argue that spirituality is intimately connected to reality and risk. That same risk can both increase awareness and also cause a person to focus on significant life-meaning.

Hugo Gryn (2000) writes of his experience as a child in Auschwitz:

> When we arrived at Auschwitz, it was a bright sunny day and a series of jet streams appeared in the sky. They may have been experimental V2 bombs, but I had not seen such a sight before, and for a while I believed that God himself would intervene... Hope was to believe that evil would be destroyed, even though it looked invincible, with no evidence whatsoever of any forces of good... And there was faith. That God knew what was happening. That he let it happen and that it had purpose. Most of the time this was difficult. Too difficult.
>
> I knew then, and know now that my survival had nothing to do with being different or better or more deserving. And one of my burdens, indeed an irrational sense of guilt ever since, has been precisely that I do not know why I survived. In all sorts of ways much of what I have tried to do and tried to be ever since has been to give some sense of meaning to that survival. (p.248)

From a child-like faith, with a strong sense of justice and feeling that God would provide retribution, Gryn moved on to a faith that placed retribution into the far future. If things were so, then God must have a plan – not one that he could understand. However, not even this made sense as the experience continued, and Gryn was forced back upon himself and upon the loneliness of that existence. He writes poignantly of being forced to write a postcard to send to relatives, only to realize that there were none left. All he was left with was the stain of the coloured pencil on his tongue.

After that, there was no simplistic meaning that Gryn could place on his experience. It was simply horrifying. Ironically, he began to discover an awareness of God in the midst of the terror, indignity and risk. Having survived that experience, like many survivors of illness such as cancer, he then had to make sense of the survival. Once again, there was no easy 'spiritual solution'. He had to live with that 'irrational sense of guilt' for the rest of his life, and to try and make sense of it.

Spirituality and religion
The stress of postmodernity and the New Age has been on moving away from the meta-narratives of religion to the idea of the individual working out their

spiritual narrative for him or herself. This has been further reinforced with the stress on spirituality in the context of health and education over the last two decades of the twentieth century. Nevertheless, it is important to explore in a little more detail how religion and spirituality do in fact relate.

As noted in Chapter 1, spirituality has most often been associated with religion. At first sight this seems reasonable since a religion is a system of faith and practice expressing a particular spirituality. Spirituality within a religious system is based in a community that has an established, corporate way of focusing upon and developing awareness of the ultimate *other*, God, as well as disciplines for ensuring that practice remains congruent with the experience of God and the religious and moral meaning that has been developed through tradition. Hence, Albin (1988, p.257) describes spirituality in the Christian religion as:

> The interaction between *doctrine, discipline, liturgy* and *life.*
>
> *Doctrine* has to do with what is believed (about the self, others, the world, and the supernatural).
>
> *Discipline* has to do with the sources of authority, the structures of corporate life and the consequences of deviant behaviour.
>
> *Liturgy* has to do with the corporate life of worship and praise. Music, prayer the various patterns of public rituals and worship have a major impact upon the attitudes, actions and lifestyles of the worshippers.
>
> *Life* refers to the individual lifestyle of the believer, not only in prayer, study and devotion but also at work at play and in one's involvement in society.
>
> Woven together, these four factors provide the basic pattern for understanding the fabric of any given spirituality. (p.257)

However, I would argue that spirituality is different from, and can be wider than, religion.

- Religion is focused in social institutions. As such it is concerned with the survival of the institution and with the maintenance of boundaries – not least through the defining of orthodox belief and orthopraxy. Spirituality does not have that same concern for the boundaries – indeed, because of the element of transcendence in it finds difficulty in defining boundaries. An important part of spirituality is precisely about the different, the unknown. This may simply be about the factual unknown or the personally unknown – uncertainty as to how the other will respond.

- Because of its group structures and concern for boundaries religion tends to be prescriptive, with meaning transmitted or revealed through the narrative of the community. Spirituality tends to involve the *discovery* of meaning, precisely because it involves reflection and integration of different levels of knowledge.

- Religion may provide an important motivational framework for spiritual development but this is not necessary for spirituality. As noted above, the New Age approaches show the possibility of a self-directed spirituality. Indeed, the mark of the New Age is that it fights against the institutional expression of spirituality.

- Religions are founded upon experience of the divine, that which is supernatural. Spirituality does not have to posit such an 'other', but can posit faith in other people, the environment and so on.

It is very easy to take a polarized view of religion and spirituality. Much New Age thinking see religions as irredeemably focused on control, with spirituality simply focused in freedom. Equally, many religious figures argue that spirituality without religion is individualistic and consumerist.

There is some but not the whole truth in these arguments:

- Religions' concern with the maintenance of the institution can lead to discouraging independent thinking and reflection.

- Religions' concern for orthodoxy and othropraxis has often led to attempts to control and even deny the affective side of spirituality. This has led to the development of moral and anthropological dualisms, not least in gender issues where women have been seen as largely somatic and affective while men are cognitive, and rational. This, then led on to a morally negative view of women (Ruether 1975).

- Religions' stress on orthodoxy has often led to a focus on guilt and shame, used by some religions at different times as the basis for evangelism and for control.

Spirituality in these terms has become defined in terms of doctrine and thus theology. This has led some religions to view their identity in terms of doctrine and credal statements. Hence, the great fear of those who thought differently and the inhuman treatment of heretics.

Over time the great religions have been aware of these problems, and have shown concern for renewal in order to do away with accretions of power and organization that obscured spiritual awareness. Christianity and Buddhism are examples of religions which themselves began in this way.

Furthermore religion often takes seriously the need for roots and tradition for the development of identity – thus respecting the insight of different faiths over history. Equally, it takes seriously the limitations of the individual and the need for a community to support and maintain the person in his or her spiritual search. A good community provides both a context for belonging and also enables the development of individual thinking, and thus a dialogue between the spiritual narrative of the individual and the corporate narrative of the community. Religion also stresses the insights of spirituality that involve commitment to the other including commitment to, and need for, the community that provides core meaning.

Religions argue that, in contrast to this, spirituality is primarily individualist and consumerist, with spirituality as primarily instrumentalist, i.e. for the purpose of *self* development. Being part of a community of faith enables the development of a mutuality in spiritual development. This means as much responding to the other as taking what one needs. However, this distinction does not really hold water. The view of spirituality outlined in this chapter is far from consumerist. Since it looks to the development of significant life-meaning precisely in relation to the significant communities of which one is a part. Hence, community-centred interactive spirituality can be developed around groups from the family to the workplace, even within sport (Parry, Robinson, Nesti and Watson 2007).

Religious experience

Ecstasy is often seen as *the* ultimate spiritual or religious experience since in it a person is taken out of him- or herself. It is often characterized by a strong sense of the other, which overwhelms the self. Rudolf Otto (1923) refers to this as the experience of the numinous, characterized as *mysterium tremendum* (p.56). There is a letting go of the self into the other. However, once again, this is not something that is restricted to the religious experience. The search for ecstasy can also be pursued through dance, drugs, group practices, and so on (Biggar 1997).

I would argue that there are major dangers with the view of spirituality as simply being experience of the ecstatic.

- Its whole approach is one that is disembodied. It seeks release from bodily constraints. To concentrate on that experience as the focus of spirituality actually takes away from the whole point of embodying spirituality in practice. Spirituality as explored earlier in this chapter is aiming to live *with* the constraints of the body, not be released *from* them.

- It can lead to a stress on the experience itself, and thus the danger of the experience becoming the end in itself. This leads to greater efforts to maintain the intensity of the experience, with dangers of addiction to the experience itself.

- The stress is very much upon affective knowledge. However, affective knowledge that lacks a link with the cognitive (or to the process of planning and commitment to a larger life plan or project) does not develop the richness of life-meaning as set out above.

- Stress on affective experience over and above all else can lead to a loss of the distinctiveness of the self, over against the other. (Trance dancing is a good example of the loss of self to the feeling induced by rhythm.)

The words 'holy' and 'sacred' are often associated with ecstatic experiences, and many spiritual practices, (such as meditation or worship) are specially designed to put one in touch with the 'other'. Places, people and literature are deemed to be holy or sacred – literally set apart from others. Hence, they have the feeling of being special and in certain contexts, pure. Spirituality as we have defined it above invites us to experience this sense of specialness not simply in the numinous but in all relationships, in that all relationships viewed empathically involve a sense of other and difference. This is not to deny the importance of ecstatic spiritual experience, which can enable a person to let go and so begin to involve their affective and somatic side in reflection as well as their cognitive side (Wright and Sayre-Adams 2000).

Conclusion

'Definition is a tool of rationality, an instrument which seeks to enclose. The term spiritual however, needs to remain elusive if it is not to betray its very identity' (Bellamy 1998, p.185). Bellamy's point is that 'spirituality' cannot be summed up in tight definition. Ideas such as transcendence are indeed hard to pin down. The danger of taking her point too much to heart is, however, that we end up failing to establish any clear understanding of what spirituality is at all. Spirituality thus becomes shapeless and ultimately useless. Indeed, a favourite game of theologians is to question the meaning of spirituality, suggesting that there are many meanings and that none are substantive, and concluding that the only substantive meaning can be found within the traditions of religion.

However, in this chapter I have attempted to show that it is possible to define spirituality. In my view it involves awareness and appreciation of the other, the development of capacity to respond and the development of meaning from that experience. Formal religions are particular expressions of this spirituality.

It is also important to define spirituality if we are to see how it connects to practice – and, the context of this book, in particular to care. For Enid, her spirituality was an important part of her recovery, and increasingly, as I will explore below, spirituality is being viewed as central to a successful handling of the experience of illness or distress, to well-being and to therapy (Fontana 2003; Miller 2003; Swinton 2001).

So how does all this relate to ethics? The focus on spirituality and care may give the impression that spirituality is in some way value-neutral, or instrumental. Hence, as Baird (2002) notes, it becomes easy to think in terms of spirituality acting as an ontological base from which ethical meaning can separately develop. However, even in the description of spirituality in this chapter there is already some concern for ethical values. For Gryn, there were issues about meaning and justice. For Enid there were issues about resolution between herself, her family and her church. In fact, any awareness of and response to the other involves values and ethical choice and it is to the ethical dimension of spirituality that I will now turn.

3

Spirituality and Ethics

Introduction

In this chapter I will begin to draw out the relationship between spirituality and ethics. I start by examining the case of a family responding to a medical crisis, noting how their reflections involved more than considering conventional ethics. They had to begin to work through their spirituality, and although this involved them in considering doctrine it also involved much more than this. I will then suggest how the type of spirituality outlined in Chapter 2 can form the basis for a framework of ethical reflection, involving awareness, critical hermeneutics, the negotiation of responsibility and creative response. I then conclude with a second case study, that of conjoined twins, to further draw out the spiritual context of ethical reflection.

Case Study

John was 78 and suffered from Alzheimer's disease. Formerly a professor of engineering, he had been an energetic man throughout his life until the condition overtook him. Above all, he had been very sharp intellectually, delighting in the cut and thrust of debate. Many times he had said to his wife and sons that he could not bear the thought of living like a shell. He did not want euthanasia but, in the event of a severe physical illness such as a heart attack or stroke, he said he would not want to be revived. He had signed an advance directive to this effect. In it he was quite precise that he wanted to refuse treatment if he were to suffer such a severe heart attack or stroke that would leave him incapable of relating to others in a meaningful way.

Now John's wife Grace, sons Tim and Geoff, and daughter Penny sat with a doctor in an anteroom and tried to focus on the fact the John had suffered a stroke. Grace was simply too shocked and afraid to take things in. The middle period of their marriage had been difficult. For a short time she had looked at the possibilities of starting afresh. However, Grace had stayed with John, partly out of a sense of duty. The duty had been the guiding feeling for her once John

55

began to suffer from Alzheimer's disease, and her identity had been partly formed by this sense of fulfilling her obligations.

Tim, the eldest son, felt that he had to communicate the views of his father. 'Now is the time to let go', he said. 'He wouldn't want to be kept alive as a vegetable'. For him the last two years, seeing his father in nursing care, had been painful. John was not the father he knew. Tim was like his father, with a top job focused on problem-solving. He felt that the family had lost his real father two years ago, and wanted simply to let John go.

Geoff was less sure. He had come to understand a different side of his father in those years. Much of his life he had feared John's intellect and felt that he would never live up to the expectations put upon him. Since his father had been in nursing care he had learned to communicate with him in a non-cognitive way and had been glad to care for him. Typically he would sit with his father holding his hand. Sometimes this would be a passive action. Sometimes it would be almost a test of strength and wrestling. If there was a chance that the effects of the stroke might be reversed Geoff wanted to keep John alive. In all this he was reinforced by his evangelical Christian faith. He believed that it was wrong to take life and this would constitute just such an action. He knew that his father had made a 'living will' but Geoff's pastor had suggested that these were tantamount to suicide.

Penny was the youngest child. Always confident of her position as her father's favourite she found it difficult to let go. At the same time she was very conscious of the effect of all this on the rest of the family. Perhaps most of all she worried for her mother. She felt that she needed to find a freedom but feared that it was too late for her. Penny was also a Christian, but one who believed that finding the most loving solution was the most important thing.

The doctor was young, uncertain and had many other problems to face. She was unsure how to bring this to a resolution. She was trained in medical ethics, but was finding it difficult to place this case into any of the examples they had covered. She began to move into the much more intuitive approach that she had had before that training.

The voice that was absent from this discussion was, of course, that of John himself. Tim tried to articulate his father's voice, but Geoff felt he had discovered quite another voice in his relationship. Grace was too powerless to even begin thinking about what John would have wanted.

The scene just described is one faced by many people everyday. It is, in one sense, simple. A decision needs to be made about whether treatment should or should not be given for a heart attack or stroke, and the family has to work through the inevitable loss of a husband and father. The only questions to be answered are when and how he will leave them. The traditional ethical tools (including deontological and utilitarian ethics) might seem adequate for making such decisions, and those are the tools that are used by the family. However, the first problem is that they do not all agree.

As a Christian, Geoff was clear that it was wrong to take life. He followed a traditional deontological view of ethics, which suggests that there are certain moral principles that are inviolable, one such being respect for human life (John Paul II 1995). Behind this basic principle were a series of beliefs that Geoff felt strongly. One was the doctrine that man was made in the image of God. Hence, human beings are sacred. To allow his father's life to be ended by not giving him treatment would be a lack of respect for his sacredness. Tied to this was a belief in the sovereignty of God – God is ruler of all and it is for Him to give and take away life. In his father's case this meant for Geoff that all efforts should be made to achieve recovery. For Geoff, therefore, doctrine led straightforwardly to an ethical conclusion.

Penny was also a Christian, but held the opposite view. As the two began to talk, Penny did two things – question the doctrinal foundation of Geoff's view, and offer a different approach to ethics. The connection between doctrine and ethics had always seemed straightforward to Geoff and Penny's challenge was the first time he had ever questioned it. Penny could not understand what the sovereignty of God was about. If God was really in charge of everything and we had to leave it to Him to 'take' her father why did we bother with medical assistance in the first place. Surely, any medical assistance that prevented death was interfering with God's sovereignty. In any case, if man was made in God's image couldn't this mean that man was given sovereignty, at least in the sense of the capacity to decide about life and death. Wasn't man a partner in all this? For Penny, however, what was worse than these points was the very idea that God was in charge of our destiny, that He knew when our time to die was and that we should leave that to Him. If that were the case why do some die and others do not? Why do some young children die in agony?

Penny was questioning the ethical basis of a doctrine that was dear to Geoff. This was not an abstruse discussion about God's power and the problem of evil. For Penny these were real issues that she faced in her job as a criminal lawyer as well as her role as a daughter. As a Christian she was also concerned about the kind of God Geoff's doctrine seemed to portray. To explain God's sovereignty in a world of suffering and inequity seemed to require that he had a plan somewhere that would ultimately justify the way in which people died, a plan that none of us are privy to. But this would point to a God who caused suffering in order to fulfil his plans.

For Penny this had two problems. First, suffering, even the most intense, was thereby considered secondary to some idea of the good, and she simply could not see how suffering could be rationalized in this way. Second, and even more difficult for her, this doctrine seemed to reveal a God who was more interested in the idea of the good than in the feelings and experience of human beings – a God who was therefore distant and had no sense of empathy.

In a very short while Penny and Geoff's doctrinal discussion had moved from respect for life and the sovereignty of God to the nature of God and the problem of evil. Yet these were not academic discussions but real discussions about how they would respond together to their father.

The result of them for Penny was to make Geoff clarify what he meant by respect for life since he seemed to be arguing that respect for life meant that they had to keep their father alive, come what may. However, for her the idea of such respect did not have any direct and obvious meaning. For her, what mattered was the immense feelings that she had for father, of care and concern, and how she would work through these was not something that could be predetermined. She felt that respect for her father meant accepting that his life was close to its end and enabling that end in the most dignified way possible. She even suggested a parallel in Jesus' end on the cross, arguing that when Jesus bowed his head (John 19: 30) this was a positive ending to his life that he was controlling.

At this point Tim began to join in the conversation. He had little interest in religion but he felt he understood something about respect. He was an engineer like his father and, as such, felt most at home ethically in utilitarian thinking – deciding what was right by calculating the greatest good for the greatest number. For Tim this was attractively practical and he could see only good coming out of allowing his father to die – it would allow his mother to move on, would distribute wealth to the family, and bring peace to his father. Geoff quickly identified this as a secular point of view, lacking any appreciation or deeper understanding of his father and the family.

But Tim argued that the distinction between the secular and the religious was of little interest to him. He felt that you could still argue from his standpoint and be religious, and in any case all the religious stuff was really in fact all about Geoff and Penny, and their needs. What they were missing, Tim felt, was consideration of other people's needs and above all of the needs of their father. If they really cared about respect, he argued, then they needed to respect his wishes and autonomy – which he had made very clear both in the way that he lived his life, in his conversation about not wanting to live like a vegetable, and in the statement that he had made as a living will. A living will or advance directive may not have the weight of law behind it but, he argued, it does have the weight of morality (Kendrick and Robinson 2002). Respect in this situation, Tim felt, was not about some theological idea, but about respecting their father's rights and wishes.

At this point, Geoff became very uncertain. He felt under real pressure but was equally determined not to let go of his position. He felt that this would be a betrayal of his beliefs, but also oddly a betrayal of his father. Geoff had always felt unsure about his father. For much of his early life he had felt that he did not measure up to his father's high standards. His father was proud of his own profession, both as a teacher and an engineer. Geoff's elder brother had followed him into civil engineering practice and had been responsible for many creative projects. Geoff, on the other hand, had spent a long time deciding what to do with his life and eventually settled on social work, something his father did not view as being a proper profession. With the onset of Alzheimer's disease all this had changed. Geoff had now been faced by a non-judgemental man who seemed to be at peace in his now reduced world. For the first time in their lives they had communicated, mostly through touch. This enabled both to express emotions, through smiles and tears. He had found a new peace with his father and found that hard to let go. For him, respect for this father was not now based on his experience of the old father, but upon the new acceptance he had found. But for Tim his father was, in effect, dead because they had sparked well together before the onset of the Alzheimer's. Intellectually and dynamically they were as one. With the onset of this disease, Tim felt that he lost his father.

Grace had so far not really contributed to the discussion. This was partly because the children were trying to shield her from it. However, she was also finding it very difficult to focus. Like Tim she felt she had lost her husband two years ago and this had been a mixed experience for her. John had been dominant in their marriage and in some ways it was a release to find the space to begin to explore life alone. At the same time there was a great sense of duty that remained. She had felt a failure when he finally went into a nursing home. She went to see him everyday, and duty had begun to provide the basis for her sense of purpose. She felt responsible for him completely. Now that she was faced by the possibility of him dying she felt that she was responsible for this, that she had not protected him adequately. Grace believed that the family was at the heart of her faith in life and this meant she had to fulfil her role as a wife.

Several things became clear through the family discussion:

- Simple resorting to classical ethical approaches (such as deontological and utilitarian ethics) did not get them very far in responding to the situation.

- Ethical positions are influenced by beliefs. In some cases this involves religious doctrines about humanity and God. In other cases it is beliefs about family or professional identity and how that affects conduct.

- Beneath, and connected to, these levels of spirituality were strong emotional issues about the family's individual relationships with John and what these meant. Sometimes these underlying emotional issues reinforce or are reinforced by the doctrines. Sometimes, however, conflicts in values emerge at several levels. At a cognitive doctrinal level there were conflicts between the views of Geoff and Penny, each eventually taking a different view of what 'respect' meant. That value conflict was further worked on when Tim entered the debate about respect and autonomy. There were also affective value conflicts occurring between Geoff and Tim around their view of John. These were both about what they valued in the relationships and about how they handled letting go of that relationship. For Geoff the affective meaning and cognitive doctrinal meaning were reinforcing each other, though they were making very different points. Grace did not have a strong cognitive doctrinal sense but she did have both a strong sense of family and familial duty – something that came from her mother – and as a result experienced a strong sense of guilt about not living up to that standard.

Also, mixed in with this discussion were important elements of religious doctrine, cultural views of the family, and family emotional and relational dynamics – all of which affected the identity of the family, the identity of the different members, and their beliefs and values. Thus, any decision was not just about the rights and wrongs of withdrawing treatment. It was about, and would thus affect, the identity and life-meaning of all involved. It became clear that all members of the family had their own different spiritualities. All members had developed life-meaning from several different communities, not just religion, and those all informed their spirituality.

In the end the decision took three days to make, not least because the family needed to check out their feelings with other people. Tim and Penny needed to hear the views of their spouses. Geoff needed to hear the views of his pastor. To his surprise, his pastor did not see this as an issue of principle, but more about the right way of letting go. Grace saw the hospital chaplain three times in three days. He was the nearest thing to the parish priest who married Tim and his wife, a positive and empowering person. At first she wanted to evade the responsibility of making a decision and pass this on to the doctor. She was also unsure about sharing her feelings with the family believing that they would disapprove of her and see her as a failure.

Tim wanted to decide quickly and take responsibility on behalf of the whole family. However, at the end of three days all the family met and shared the responsibility for choosing to withdraw treatment. None of this was a magical or miraculous development. It was simply the result of a group of people working hard to make sense of their shared experience and to make the response that was right for them. At the heart of this was the ultimate 'other' – the experience of death and loss, something that no-one can make sense of before it happens. Wisely, the doctor and chaplain had not tried to rush them but have given them space to articulate their thoughts and feelings, their spiritualities and to work out how they would fulfil their responsibilities. In the process they had begun to work out their responsibilities not just to John but to each other and to themselves. This meant Geoff letting go, Tim stepping back a little, and Grace letting her children into her fears and hopes. None of this took away from their ongoing dynamics and problems but it did help them to make the decision and it did give them a basis from which to continue working together after the funeral.

The spiritual framework of ethics

This case study points to the complex relationship that exists between spirituality and ethics – one that I will now explore through the three headings suggested in the last chapter: awareness, developing life-meaning and creative response.

Awareness

If existential awareness of the other is central to spirituality it is also critical for ethics. At one level one could see awareness simply as a neutral activity about gathering data in order to be fully aware of a situation and to be in a position to make an ethical decision. There is no doubt that it *is* important to be sure of the data. However, such an approach assumes that the data for an ethical situation is objective and that all we need to do is gather it. Although such an approach acknowledges the need to work with other stakeholders to do this

(Robinson 2002), it seems confident that ultimately we will find out what the facts of the case are.

However, as Spohn (1997) suggests, there is no value-free awareness of any situation, 'We make choices in the world that we notice, and what we notice is shaped by the metaphors and the habits of the heart that we bring to experience' (p.116). In other words, perception is always conditioned by the values and beliefs that we hold implicitly or explicitly. A good example of this is the parable of the rich man in Luke 16:20–27 (New English Bible).

> There was once a rich man, who dressed in purple and the finest linen, and feasted in great magnificence every day. At his gate, covered with sores, lay a poor man named Lazarus, who would have been glad to satisfy his hunger from the scraps from the rich man's table. Even the dogs used to come and lick his sores. One day the poor man died and was carried away by the angels to live with Abraham. The rich man also died and was buried, and in Hades where he was in torment he looked up; and there far away was Abraham with Lazarus close beside him. 'Abraham, my father' he called out, 'take pity on me!'... But Abraham said 'Remember my child that all the good things fell to you while you were alive, and all the bad to Lazarus; now he has his consolation here and it is you who are in agony. But that is not all: there is a great chasm fixed between us; no one from our side who wants to reach you can cross it, and none may pass from your side to us.'

What is perhaps most interesting about this parable is that fact that the rich man finds himself separated from God because of his lack of awareness of the poor man, and of his needs. The rich man is not purely evil, because he subsequently asks if his brothers can be warned about all this, so they can avoid his fate. He looks at the problem, and accepts it is a problem, as simply a lack of awareness. Hence, he wants his brothers to be made aware. But Abraham then tells him that not even the appearance of a supernatural figure will make them aware. No one simply lacks awareness. Our awareness is conditioned by what we find important, our beliefs and values. Furthermore, we are responsible for the values and beliefs that we hold. Hence, it is not that the rich man simply lacked awareness of the poor man, but rather that he chose to be aware of other things, based around the values of wealth and security. His awareness was conditioned by his beliefs and values.

Murdoch (1972) develops this theme around a generic spirituality. She argues that everyday moral vision is egocentric and that in order for that to be widened we need to transcend our perceptions. This means being able to transcend our thoughts and feelings – what we bring from our past to the perceptions of the present. Murdoch suggests that there needs to be connection to some transcendent source of goodness and beauty in order for this to happen. For her this was something like Plato's 'Form of the Good', a transcendent ideal.

However, Murdoch's model focuses perhaps too much on the conceptual. What prevents someone from standing back from thoughts and feelings is often deeply held beliefs operating at an affective level around personal relationships that have established a sense of identity. A person, for example, may have based their ethical meaning around the feeling she has for her partners or parents, looking primarily to please them. Moving beyond that needs more than a Platonic ideal, and more than just a technique to develop spiritual awareness.

Levinas (1998), Bauman (1989) and Baird (2002) take this further, suggesting that ethical commitment – that is, responsibility – to the other precedes awareness. In this view ethics would be at the heart of, and indeed precede, spirituality. These three writers develop spirituality in different ways in response to the experience of the Holocaust. For them it is not simply a matter of developing spirituality such that we can achieve transcendence – to see the situation and thus respond better. Instead, they propose that it is not possible to develop that spiritual awareness without an ethical commitment to the other: spirituality begins with a sense of responsibility to the other. Without that sense of prior responsibility we cannot begin to see the other in an inclusive way.

This means, however, genuinely seeing the other in all their ambiguity, their sameness, their difference, their good and their bad. For Levinas this even applies to the oppressors, such as the perpetrators of the Holocausts. Unless we begin with responsibility for other, then some, by omission or commission, will be excluded from our view of humanity – and that way lies the Holocaust. For Levinas this places the face of the other at the heart of the ethical obligation. The physical presence of the other in his or her uniqueness calls us to care, without any reference to rights or even to rational grounds for why we should be ethical. As Baird (2002) puts it 'I am called to be responsible for the other before understanding who the other is or why I should engage with him or her ethically' (p.70). There is a similar stress in McIntyre's later work (1999) around the idea of ethics being built upon the vulnerability of the other. Here, self-transcendence does not occur through reference to some *idea* of the good but rather through the openness and response to the unique irreplaceable other. I will explore this in more detail in the next chapter. None of this precludes the possibility of finding greater awareness of the other through reaching out and becoming more aware of the divine. It simply argues that in both cases responsibility and awareness are very much tied together.

Levinas argues that the other is incommensurable – that is, cannot be summed up or contained. However, as Baird (2002) notes, if the other is totally incommensurable then he or she becomes unknowable – in effect, anonymous, whether he or she, divine or human. As I suggested in the last chapter, the other is essentially ambiguous, both different and the same – without recognizing some sameness with the other it would be impossible to be aware of them. In John's family there was immense familiarity between the members, but they were also in one sense strangers to each other and to themselves. They had previously not shared their deepest beliefs and feelings and had not seen each other in a crisis such as this. This led to seeing new things about themselves. Tim, for instance, had not realized that he was so assertive. Fasching (1992) suggests that this increased awareness of one's motivations and patterns of behaviour is critical to ethical reflection.

Throughout the three days it took to reach a decision John's family were gradually becoming more aware of each other. Although there were some pre-existing familial bonds these were not defined. In addition to their shared background there were also very different experiences from their relationships with John. Hence, they had to begin to be aware of and work through those differences and the associated needs. What sustained their work was a sense of responsibility, individual and shared. The 'face' of John and the faces of all the family called forth a response to question their beliefs and values and that demanded that they find a way of sharing responsibility. In turn, this led to working through a response to him and to each other.

Developing meaning

The family in the case of John happened to be very articulate at verbalizing their thoughts, but their attempts at making meaning went on at many levels. This was not about discovering meaning that was 'out there' but meaning that was focused in several relationships and groups. As such it was messy. Doctrinal meaning, usually focused in a worshipping community, was focused into the immediate concern and in turn was mediated through relationships and what they had shown about value and belief. The meaning of the situation needed to be experienced at cognitive, affective, somatic and relational levels, with the affective and somatic sometimes fuelling the conceptual/doctrinal levels. Certainly any idea of faith, hope and purpose was mediated through relationships. The two sons had both in different ways bought up in a conditional view of value – their value was conditional on fulfilling their father's expectations, as they perceived them. Both Geoff and Tim were in their own way trying to apply ethics previously worked out into a practical situation, and as a result both were tested.

It is precisely in such situations that belief and values will be tested. It is comparatively easy to sit around a study group and discuss issues but when faced by a life-and-death matter hitherto hidden aspects of belief come close to the surface, and as they do so then the meaning and the identity of the person is tested. Geoff had been to a deanery ecumenical evening three months earlier on the subject of 'the right to die' and this had concluded that Christianity was set firmly against it. In that situation he had had no reason to question his belief and value links. Now he had cause to question them. This did not automatically mean that he would lose his faith. But, it does mean that entirely new questions arise, precisely because of the personal relationships that affect that ethical identity. In different ways then this points us towards considering a system of ethics in which underlying spiritual meaning is constantly tested and critiqued as a matter of course.

CRITICAL HERMENEUTICAL ETHICS

Don Browning (2006) suggests that such an ethics can be built around the work of Ricoeur (1982) and Gadamer (1982). They argue that we begin ethics with a basic and general hope for the good things of life. Just what that assertion might mean only becomes clear as we relate to particular groups, such as family, schools, business, or religion. These groups provided tested meaning and practice to show what is right.

Inevitably because of the plurality of existence – be that the plural self (Taylor 1989), or communities that embody plurality – there will be conflicts of value, tested by events and leading to the questioning of accepted goods. Browning's description of this (2006) seems to assume that such conflicts will be exceptional, but in this I would differ from him. First, such conflict is common at point of crisis and transition, both in terms of individual development and change, and in major emotional or physical trauma (Bridges 1980). Second, such conflicts are also common in corporate experience, not least when major changes occur in a company. Much management of change is about dealing with values and a view of purpose and meaning in relationships.

Nonetheless, the basic idea still applies and Browning (2006) suggests that any conflict will set one exploring the 'deeper integration of our conventional practices' (p.9). This is very much an interpretative process that looks at the classic conventional texts. This might range from a profession's statement of purpose and code of practice to the stories and codes in religious texts. Such texts, argues Browning, are not just to be internalized, they must also be critiqued. Critique in this sense involves looking at the conventional position and asking if the insights are 'valid and lasting' and if they can be applied in different cultures. At the heart of this critique is dialogue with others in that situation. This is a critique not simply of the texts, and stories of the community but also the way in which that community had grown and the way in which the stories and codes were used. This fits in with the view of the religious group, for instance, as always reforming itself. In all this, values are not found simply in texts but also in emotions and in practice.

It is important to see this critical hermeneutic as a part of what it is to reflect ethically. I would only add to Browning's restatement of Ricoeur's view that it needs to go beyond a focus on disciplines such as theology and psychology. First, there is the critique of particular doctrines, which come from a cognitive perspective. However, critique of doctrines (as the liberation theologians have shown us) is more than analysis of concepts. It also looks at the way in which we use concepts, and in particular at the ways that we use doctrine to further any power arrangements. This includes wrestling with established meaning of tradition noted by Fasching and Dechant (2001).

The second level of critiques is much more difficult. This involves reflection on the affective content of spirituality and may involve questioning ethical identity. In the case of John's family this involved looking at the psychological dynamic and their associated values that held in place different people's views of the situation. This level of critique is much more painful and difficult to engage in. This is the level of wrestling with people and groups that embody traditions, our literal 'forefathers' that Fleischacker (1994) sees as being at the base of any psychological and cultural development. Without such wrestling there is little chance of moving into an epistemic distance – a distance that is necessary to know the other. Too great a psychological distance or too close a one can obscure our understanding of the other. Both Tim and Geoff found that their values were held in place by their relationships with their father, and to reach a decision that they could live with they had to find a certain distance from their father in order to see and hold both his bad and good sides. A core element of this was around the fact that John had been the ground of faith in different ways for his family. Working through their relationship with him meant working at that faith, along with faith in family, professional identity and God.

There are many psalms that show vivid examples of this kind of wrestling.

How long, O Lord? Wilt thou forget me forever?

How long will thou hide thy face from me?

How long must I bear pain in my soul

And sorrow in my heart all the day? (Psalm 13, vv.1–2)

The psalmist here is continuing to show faith in God, because he continues to talk to him, while at the same time questioning why God seems to have deserted him in his suffering. In effect, he is questioning the ground of faith. This is not questioning simply the doctrine of God but God himself. Brueggemann (1984) writes that this is an act of boldness in that it 'insists that all such experiences of disorder are a proper subject for discourse with God' (p.93).

The third level of critique involves examination of practice, and how that relates to doctrine and faith. This critique of integrity is precisely what Tim fired off against his Christian siblings. Communities, relationships and related doctrines frame our ethical meaning, but they will always have limitations and thus will always need to be critiqued. Hence, this attempt to critique becomes a critical part of ethical awareness and knowledge. We know and learn through critique.

At the heart of any critical dynamic is difference and plurality, and this demands dialogue. Difference and plurality is not an added ethical extra that can be examined once one has sorted out the moral meaning. Ethical plurality, in fact, is often thought to be a problem for ethics – leading to ethical relativism, and the breakdown of shared ethical meaning. However, I will now argue that difference and plurality are central to the development of ethical meaning. There are three reasons for this.

First, we learn from difference. Only when we come up against the other, outside or inside the community, do we begin to question our prejudgement – something we all have because that is how we learn, by modifying our view of the world. Markham (1994) highlights how this occurs in the interfaith world. This learning involves three aspects. By being faced with other perspectives we have to *articulate* our own perspectives. For many this might be the first time of actually voicing one's own ethical position, and thus the first time hearing one's own thoughts out loud. Difference, in turn, then *tests* one's ethical perspective, and forces one to begin to justify it. Finally, difference reveals both partiality and possibility, the limitations of one's own expressions and the possibilities beyond that – new perspectives to illuminate us. All this can emerge from dialogue with the other, which takes in values, doctrine and relationships.

Second, plurality is good. Looking at the Holocaust, Bauman (1989) argues that ethical plurality is precisely what prevents the imposition of an overarching view-point. There is some truth in this. He focuses in his mighty book *Modernity and the Holocaust* on the experiments of Stanley Milgram (2005). Milgram's famous psychological experiments would not have got through today's research ethics committees – and yet his experiments have proved most enlightening, and recently popular in academic circles (Bauman 1989 and Zimbardo 2007) and in the media. Milgram set out to examine the clash between authority and individual conscience. His participants were told that they were involved in an experiment about reinforcing learning with pain, which would involve them administering electric shocks to a learner, whenever an incorrect response was made. They were encouraged by authority figures to give more and more powerful shocks. The learner was in fact an actor, and the shocks were only feigned. Analysis of this and other experiments revealed that between 61 and 66 per cent of participants were prepared to give increasingly powerful shocks until they were ready to cause death, when ordered to do so by figures of authority. Bauman (1989) suggests that only the conscious articulation of different beliefs and judgements will guard against slipping into the response of the research participants, avoiding taking responsibility for the other. He concludes: 'A most remarkable conclusion flowing from the full set of the Milgram experiments is that pluralism is the best preventative medicine against morally normal people engaging in morally abnormal actions' (p.165).

Third, plurality and difference can also be said to be the key to the ethical endeavour. Dealing with plurality and difference requires more than just a critical appreciation of different values but also awareness and appreciation of the other who is the bearer of those values. It is not simply a conceptual exercise or an attempt to provide a solution to a problem, or an exercise in developing rules for dialogue, as in Habermas's discourse ethics (Habermas 1992). It is also not simply a tolerance of difference, but rather an engaging with difference in practice. It involves relating to the other, and therefore requires commitment to the other. This forces us back on to an ethics that is not founded primarily on rules or principles but on the responsibility for the self and other, and the working out of that responsibility.

RESPONSIBILITY NEGOTIATIONS

A natural consequence of increasing spiritual awareness is an increased awareness of the needs of the other, and thus of their moral demand upon the self. Issues of how responsibility will be fulfilled arise naturally. Finch and Mason (1993) suggest that it is precisely this area of responsibility negotiation that provides the testing moment for any moral response, and that for the most part it is through this process that families begin to address ethical issues. Their research found that the negotiation of actual practice was effective at providing shared moral meaning in families that had no ethical rules or even vocabulary for such rules. The negotiation itself was the means whereby the shared images of individuals within the family were transmitted from one situation to the next. This formed the basis of a moral reputation, such that 'people were being constructed and reconstructed as moral beings' (p.170). The negotiations that they describe (such as how a family will share care of an elderly relative) tended to be built on previous work, often decades old, and most often leading to a confirmation or development of the previous practice. Their work points to a critical element of moral reflection which is often not given due weight precisely because formal principles are not always part of the process. These, nonetheless, might easily be drawn from reflection on the practice.

The major problem with this is not the negotiation *per se* but rather that the negotiation which they describe did not easily accommodate challenge or change. Hence, in the central case which they use we see different members of the family being confirmed in their responsibilities, but no development of genuine collaborative practice. One adult child is left to care for their widowed mother, and the other two accept the moral identity of their sibling and refuse to take responsibility for care in the event of him not being able to fulfil it. Hence, the activity described by Finch and Mason actually seems more like consultation, in which there is communication and acceptance of intentions, with no space for the challenge of mutual responsibility.

Negotiation in fact involves:

- Clarifying the situation and the need. Helping all involved to define and establish the need, and the shared responsibility to respond.

- Analysing the stakeholders, those who have a concern or interest. This includes assessing stakeholder resources and limitations.

- Analysing how responsibility is fulfilled now. This can involve looking at those who are taking too much or too little responsibility.

- Working out how responsibility can be shared more effectively, and planning around that.

Working through that involves development of identity. In the case study in this chapter, Tim, for instance, perceived himself as taking most responsibility for his father in recent years. He visited his father, and acted as Power of Attorney, and so on. He had not realized that Geoff and Penny had also been visiting frequently and were thus involved in John's care. When he realized this at first he saw it as a threat to his identity as the oldest child, and as a criticism of his care. As a busy successful engineer he had limited time and liked to get things done quickly. As the conversations between the siblings progressed Tim began to accept his limitations and to allow his siblings more space in the caring. In turn, his own contributions were more openly recognized and valued, giving him a much firmer sense of moral identity.

Creative response

Even having worked through all the different relationships and their meaning it is not possible to end up with a simple decision that this or that action is morally right. Once responsibility has been negotiated then the person has become identified with the response and an ethical response calls for change, personal involvement and possibly a shared project. Change may occur in response to the situation, and for Grace, certainly, there had to be change. The man who had been very much the ground of her faith, with whom she had found purpose, had now gone and she had to begin to find new meaning in her life. This change might be in having to reconcile different and conflicting values. Geoff found that many of his religious values were up for questioning and he began to learn to place relationships at the centre of his values rather than principles. The change here could involve reconciling relationships, something that Geoff and Tim began to focus on.

The family then had to put these changes into practice, not just in terms of agreeing to let go of their father, but in establishing projects that would respond to and initiate change. For Geoff and Tim this meant being determined to meet more frequently. For all, it meant sharing responsibility over decision-making, which enabled the integration of a narrative unity. As Ricoeur (1992) puts it, this involves 'an integration of actions in global projects, be that in professional, community or family life' (p.180). This addresses the plurality at the heart of such communities in relation to practice and shared demands. The ethical response involves the engagement of the person in the community and in turn, this leads to both what Ricoeur calls a development in moral imagination, and a development and extension of that community. Hence, at the heart of this stage is creative and transformative response. In effect, this involves the creation of good *in* practice, quite the opposite of application of 'the good' to practice. As Gutiérrez (1988) describes it: the 'continuous creation, never ending, of new ways to be human' (p.21).

The discrete action of the continuing community by itself extends and embodies the value and belief system previously held. In effect, the creative response involves the creation and articulation of meaning. In turn, this development can have effects beyond the community. In the case of John's family this moved to the way in which the grandchildren related to Grace, and also the partners of the children.

Of course, the value and beliefs systems of all communities are by definition limited. They can only provide a limited perspective on the good that they try to embody. Hence, they have to respond continually in this creative way to show something of that good. As Bauman (1989) reminds us, 'The moral self is always haunted by the suspicion that it is not moral enough' (Bauman, p.60). A parallel can be found in the world of performing arts. As the pianist Schnabel once said of Beethoven's Hammerklavier Piano Sonata, it is always much better than it can be performed. However, we keep performing, hoping that the qualities and the spirit of that mighty score might be embodied. And the full meaning of such a score can only be found in the performing, not simply in the music theory or historical background.

In the case study about John, the doctor gave space for reflection, and in this respect had realized that what was at issue was not simply the question of whether treatment should be withdrawn. This contrasted with what the doctor had been taught in medical ethics, which would have focused on the issues of freedom and rights of the patient, best interest and how this might be defined by the doctor, and respect for life. Looking at ethics purely through such a refined lense ignores the reality that such ideas only take on meaning in the context of relationship and thus in terms of the wider spirituality of the group. Freedom to decide on treatment through living wills is important and should be respected but once people are faced by the decision to withdraw treatment then patient freedom is only one element in the decision-making. 'Best interest' from a medical point of view can bear little relationship to best interest of the community who have to make the decision. Hence, ideas such as best interest can only be worked out in the network of the patient's core relationships.

Summing up so far

We can thus begin to see a moral framework emerging from spirituality as we have outlined it so far. This involves several characteristics:

- Many traditions see spirituality has moving away from the world, transcending worldly concerns. The spiritual framework above, however, shows an openness to and involvement in that world (Baird 2002).

- Other models of spirituality view it as enabling the transcendence of the self to the ultimate horizon, often the divine. This connection to the divine enables an expanding of consciousness and thus acts as the basis of ethical awareness and responsibility. Hence, in the model of spirituality I am proposing the reaching out to the other precedes the ethics. Levinas and Baird suggest that ethics, in the sense of responsibility for the other, is at the centre of any transcendence of the self. It actually enables greater awareness. In Baird's words (2002), 'ethical responsibility is no longer to be defined as the altruistic outcome of a prior self transcending encounter with the horizon of ultimate being and meaning but is rather integral to the self-transcendence itself' (p.119). In the next chapter I will argue that it is love that is the focus of this responsibility.

- Ethical meaning has to be articulated in dialogue. Without articulation of values it is very hard to be aware of what they are or how they affect out perception. Without articulation there can be no attempt to wrestle with the doctrines or the grounds of faith – a wrestling that is broad ranging and complex, involving cognitive, affective and relational dimensions of meaning. Because of the holistic nature of its meaning, articulation involves narrative, not just analysis of values.

- Ethics is essentially a learning experience. Learning takes place at cognitive, affective and somatic levels. Hence, in our case study the family had to learn about their feelings and how these related to their beliefs and values. Damasio (1994) sets out the importance of emotional perception in all this. The learning experience examines the previous frameworks of meaning, including beliefs and values. If the creative response is one that embodies, and in so doing creates, moral and spiritual meaning then each new response is something of a learning experience. In all this the person is invited to take responsibility for that learning, which then means a constant reflection on frameworks of meaning. Hence, responsibility for reflection sits alongside responsibility for the other. If it is a learning process then there can never be any 'perfect' solution to any ethical dilemma or problem. Each response hopefully will enable further learning.

- It is worth saying that some theologies discourage this learning and responsibility. Hull (1991), for instance, notes some Christian theologies that see learning a negative thing. He suggests that the root of such theologies is in their view of a God who does not learn. Because such God is omnipotent He does not need to learn, so the argument goes, and to suggest that He does is to paint the picture of a fallible and less than perfect God. Three arguments weigh against such a view.

  ○ First, focusing purely on the Christian narratives, there is clear evidence in the Scriptures of learning. God, for instance, chooses to stop sending prophets and send his own Son. His Son tests his values and beliefs in the wilderness, and at various points makes choices that require decisions.

  ○ Second, the assertion that God is omnipotent is one that carries the assumption that perfection is quantitative – God must know all. However, the narrative suggests a God who actually allows himself to be vulnerable, open to different possibilities and relationships. In the light of that, perfection is not about knowing all before it happens, but rather about true wisdom in relationships.

  ○ Third, learning is a key part of human experience. Ignoring this dimension brings into question the reality of both the doctrines of the Incarnation and the Creation (at least in the sense of the man being made in the image of God). It might also be added that, as Hull notes, theology that devalues learning can easily be used to control communities rather than empower their members.

- The approach described in this book brings together the development of the person (taking responsibility for making meaning), and the development of community. Plurality is at the heart of both. In John's case there is the community of the family but the members are all active in more than one other community, professional, faith, cultural, other families and so on. Often the different values at the heart of each of these communities are kept quite separate, but the experience of having to respond together to the situation over John led the family to examine and challenge the different belief and values systems they held. The community that was being developed in this exchange was one that actually transcended itself, becoming aware of how it related to other groups and their values.

This view is close to Browning's view of the family (2006). He sees the family as a primary community of commitment, whose circle is gradually widened to take in other commitments. The case above, however, suggests greater complexity. First, the family has plural views within it, which test out the commitment of the family members if working together as a whole and enables the members to develop their personal commitment to the family as a whole and to their father. Second, the spirituality of the family is worked out in response to a radical challenge. This brings together these plural perspectives, but also makes the members find the meaning of their commitment, something that had not been there for many years. Third, the plural family community also reflected a plural religious community. Penny and Geoff were committed Christians, and Grace found echoes of a former faith through her conversations with the chaplain. The experience of John's stroke revealed for them a spirituality that was much broader than their religious communities. Geoff, for instance, thought that his spirituality was summed up in his church, but in fact it also involved his family and their diverse narratives. To his surprise, moreover, he discovered that his core ground of faith was his father, and not his church, and this relationship had to be addressed first. Meaning, then, for the family members, including faith, hope and purpose, was based in several different groups, and had to be worked through at cognitive, affective, and somatic levels. What brought that plurality of meaning together was the shared experience and the shared response in practice.

The stress on plurality as being central to the ethical endeavour reminds one of Bakhtin's idea of polyphonic truth. 'Truth reveals when one can hear and comprehend both or all voices simultaneously, and more than that, when one's voice joins in creating something similar to a musical chord. In a chord, voices remain different, but they form a different kind of music, which is in principle unachievable by a single voice' (Sidorkin 1999, p.30).

Truth comes from the many voices forming a 'chorus' (Bakhtin 1984, p.71). One might legitimately ask what constitutes the authoritative discourse in all this. In Browning's terms this is about how we recognize the authority of the community, such that while making any critique of it we are still to remain as a part of that community. I will return to that question in the final chapter.

Ethics in the case of conjoined twins

A case study such as that of John and his family could be seen as purely a pastoral one (i.e. by those who prefer to avoid the ethical dimension of pastoral care in favour of focusing on the unconditional care). Yet it does carry a significant ethical dimension and should therefore be treated as such. Often in a busy hospital a doctor will advise a family in one way or the other and not give them time to think and feel the occasion as being one of significance. For most families, however, such decisions are likely to be one of the major decisions they will take in their whole life history. It is therefore very important that they be given the space to work through that history and its meaning.

As a contrast to that case study I will now briefly consider a case study that is primarily seen as 'ethical' – that of conjoined twins – and show how this, too, involved a spiritual dimension.

Case study

The case involved Jodie and Mary (pseudonyms), born conjoined to parents on the island of Gozo in Summer 2000. It became clear that both twins could not survive together and that if the two were separated then the weaker one, Mary, would die, partly because she depended upon the respiratory system of Jodie. As Simon Lee (2003) notes, this case created massive public concern when the hospital in Manchester that was dealing with the twins recommended that the two be separated in order to give Jodie the chance of life. What followed was a very public ethical debate when the parents appealed against the medical decision to operate. This debate was mostly carried out between the courts who were appealed to and the Roman Catholic Church. The former dealt in case law and attempted to find cases analogous to this one. The latter dealt in broad principles. Neither approach was wholly adequate. The Church, through the submission of the Cardinal Archbishop of London, set out the following arguments:

1. Human life is sacred. This was seen as an inviolable principle that one should never intend to end an innocent person's life by omission or commission.

2. A person's 'bodily integrity' should not be invaded when the consequences to that person involve neither benefit nor harm.

3. There is no duty to preserve life if the preservation of that life involves a grave injustice to another. Hence, he argued that the grave injustice of taking life away from Mary made the preservation of Jodie's life unacceptable.

4. There is no duty to preserve life if extraordinary means have to be used.

5. The natural authority of the parents should be accepted and their rights only overridden if there is clear evidence that they are acting contrary to what is owed to their children.

The judges accepted the first four principles but came to exactly the opposite conclusion: that respect for life was best expressed in allowing Mary to die.

Lee suggested that the conflict was not so much between different values as one found *within* such broad values. When faced by a case such as this the broad values admit of different and conflicting outcomes.

For their part the judges argued by analogy and precedent, offering several comparable cases. One such in the USA involved conjoined twins where the parents agreed to have a similar operation within a short time of the medical team asking for their permission. Rabbi and priest were present to advise. Deeply religious Jews, they refused to make a decision without the guidance of their rabbi. Some of the hospital staff also refused to be involved until advice from Christian priests had been sought. Rabbis and priests were both present to advise and all agreed that it was permissible and based their own judgement on analogies. One, for instance, involved the scenario of two men jumping from a plane. The parachute of one does not open and he clings on to the first man. His parachute cannot support both of them. The rabbis agreed that it was permissible for the first man to kick the other away as the man whose parachute did not open was already 'designated' for death.

However, none of the analogies fitted the conjoined twins situation exactly, and certainly none could address the views of the Archbishop. Lee notes that several doctrines seemed to underlay the principles set out in this case. In particular, there was a theological anthropology that sets out human as being both uniquely valuable and also interdependent. Once again, however, this does not begin to offer a solution. The doctrine and principles, rather, provide a framework of meaning in which the tragic experience could be explored.

The Christian contribution was important but limited the reflection on spirituality to doctrine. Moreover, it had had a particular perspective and moral identity, including a felt responsibility for maintaining moral truth and practice in the future. Hence, some of the arguments used were analogous to those used in the debate about abortion. This was especially used to address the concern that if this action was accepted in the case of Mary and Jodie it could lead to a slippery slope. This argument runs something like, 'we must maintain a moral standard now or this will lead to a desensitization of practitioners, such that in the future they will allow this to happen without genuine reflection'. Lee suggests that such an argument is fallacious. It points to the danger of something where there is no evidence that it will happen.

This case also raises the issue of negotiation of responsibility and the parents. Some commentators have suggested that the dynamics of the situation might have involved the parents trying to shift responsibility for the decision from themselves on to the church or the medical team. This then raises the issue as to whose responsibility it was to decide and whether the parents should have been given more support, such as counselling, to help them work through the meaning of what was happening and so find some hope in the situation. It could equally be argued that the decision was so difficult that it was necessary to share responsibility. The whole process could be seen as an opportunity to work through that responsibility and how it should be shared.

Spirituality can involve working through to a happy ending, but just as often is about finding meaning in the experience of tragedy. At the core was the simple tragedy that at least one girl was bound to die. The sense of tragedy experienced by the parents must have been intense: the loss of one or both of their daughters, the feeling of guilt and impotence at not being able to solve this problem and the feeling of uncertainty as to how this might be seen by the church. However, during the actual process real care was taken to listen to all the different views presented and the judges were therefore very sensitive about the church perspective. However, as Lee suggests, there could have been more time spent on reflecting on and refining the views and feelings of all the different stakeholders, especially the parents, and how they might begin to find meaning in the tragedy.

Whilst a full spirituality did not seem to have been worked through in this case, it is nonetheless a good example of how different parties can work together to wrestle with beliefs and values in a very public way. The reasons why I argue this are as follows.

- The debate was so sensitive that there was no polarization into secular or spiritual/religious views. At the heart of it was a strong sense of commitment to all parties. There was no sense of a simple divide between law and ethics, and all parties explored belief and values, brought together in the need to respond to tragedy.

- As all parties tried to work through the truth about the situation there was the basis of a critical hermeneutical approach. Spirituality and values were articulated and illustrated by all participants and their meaning was tested in the situation. Precisely, because of this underlying concern about the family there was no attempt to make this a knock-down philosophical argument. Spirituality and values were not seen as being exclusively owned by any one group. Hence, it was acceptable for judges and the church to test and challenge each others' interpretation of all the values and principles. Taken in this light it is a good example of wrestling with something that went beyond boundaries – whether religious, spiritual or philosophical.

- As I have suggested, there were major issues about responsibility and responsibility negotiation, both in terms of responsibility for the actual decision and also responsibility for publicly addressing belief and values in practice. In the event these were shared.

- As Lee (2003) notes, this was a learning experience for all involved. Because all the different perspectives were taken into account, this enabled a change in the understanding of the moral imperatives. The very idea of the 'common good', underlying much of the religious input in this case gives space for such change, precisely because it does not aim to impose some worked out view of the good but looks to give men and women 'the freedom to assume responsibility for their own lives' (p.47).

Lee (2003) sums up the dynamics in this way. It is possible to argue:

- that it was right for the parents to stake out their position

- that the doctors were entitled to challenge their decision

- that it was right, given some public criticism of the parents' standpoint, the challenge from the doctors and the decision by the first instance judge (who was deciding against the parents without the benefit of all the arguments which the Court of Appeal later heard), for the Archbishop to articulate the overarching moral considerations

- that it was permissible nonetheless for the judges to apply this framework, or their own variation on its themes, to reach a different conclusion

- that the best reasoning to defend such a decision has yet to be formulated

- that we are all therefore learning from this uneasy case (p.47).

Conclusion

In both the cases in this chapter, spirituality, in its broadest sense, has been central to ethical reflection and response. Perhaps most importantly it has been worked through in a public or semi-public way. The spiritual meaning was not left to the individual to work through in private but was addressed through dialogue with others. From this I have concluded that:

- Spirituality provides a framework for ethical reflection and response.

- Ethics, in the sense of responsibility for the other, precedes spirituality.

- Responsibility for the other actually enables the development of spiritual awareness.

- Ethics, in the sense of responsibility for the other is also deepened by self-transcendent awareness. The example I gave was of greater awareness of the divine. However, it could be equally be true that greater existential awareness of the environment, for instance, could lead to a deepened ethical response. The case of global warming is one current example of this.

- Ethics and spirituality involve a continual wrestling with tradition and narratives. At the heart of this is narrative and dialogue, which involve mutual challenge. This differs markedly from the dynamic of ethics simply flowing from a belief system. Because of the plurality within and between communities as well as the limitations of any community, this critical hermeneutic is an inevitable feature of ethics.

- Spirituality, in the sense of identity, is worked out through the development of a person's responsibility for the beliefs and values that they adhere to, through the negotiation of responsibility for the other and through planning and implementation of a creative response. This is transformative of the self and the community, thus embodying new meaning. In all this, new challenges and changes question, but do not drive, spirituality. Rather spirituality engages with and enables creative and collaborative change.

Mustakova-Possardt (2004) sums up much of this in the idea of critical moral consciousness. This is characterized by 'a deepening life-long integration of moral motivation, agency and critical discernment' (p.245). The bedrock for this, she suggests, is both an integrated sense of moral identity and moral understanding of the interdependence of life. Along with that is a 'critical historical capacity to differentiate authentic moral authority from other dominant forms of authority' (p.255).

The approach to spirituality that I am advocating moves away from the dualism that sees beliefs and values as being separate domains, or a one-way relationship of values emerging from beliefs. It also breaks away from the simplistic division of process and content in ethics. Some would argue that the content of ethics is primary and that process is really of secondary importance. The framework and process suggested above in fact embodies ethical content, and in and through the quality of the response further reveals ethical meaning.

It could, of course, be argued that this is really the assertion of a normative spirituality, one which therefore takes away from the autonomy of the individual. I go on to examine the idea of autonomy later, arguing that my view of spirituality actually develops and deepens it. However, there tend to be certain core values in spirituality, and lined against them is what might be termed sin. Sin in this context is not to do with moral judgement about discrete actions, but rather with lack of engagement with spirituality, involving:

- a lack of awareness of the other, which in turn, can lead to fragmentation and alienation

- a lack of awareness of value and beliefs and how they relate to practice

- the distortion of reality, or the unquestioning acceptance of reality as 'given'

- the denial or distortion of responsibility. Distortion might involve taking on too much or too little responsibility
- the denial of hope, other than in the self or the immediate group.

It is perhaps important to note here that this denial, fragmentation, alienation and distortion does not arise simply from a lack of reflection. It can arise precisely from reflection that is limited by the values and beliefs already held. It is thus ultimately a matter of choice on our part. For most, the choice is not simply rational, and the moment of making it is buried deep in the subconscious. However, as I will suggest in Chapter 6, successful therapy does enable that choice to be recognized and then a new one to be made. For others, the choice is made for them by the group, an extreme example being that of the Third Reich. We tend to think of the Third Reich as being innately unspiritual. Yet, as Burleigh (2000) shows, it was in fact built upon a series of quasi-religious beliefs and practices. Moreover, these were the object of frequent reflection expressed in ritual. What led the Third Reich into alienation was precisely its intentional denial of any 'other' beyond their group, and the associated denial of a plurality of views within the community.

So what enables Mustakova-Possardt's critical moral consciousness, and what provides its moral content? For that we must turn to love – the subject I consider in the next chapter.

4

Love

When the Pharisees heard that [Jesus] had silenced the Sadducees they came together. And one of them, a lawyer, asked him a question to test him. 'Teacher, which is the greatest commandment in the law?' And he said to him, 'You shall love the Lord your God with all your heart, and with all your soul, and with all your mind.' This is the greatest and first commandment. And the second is like it, 'You shall love your neighbour as yourself. On these commandments hang all the law and the prophets.'

(Matthew 22: 34–40)

Speak of me as I am; nothing extenuate,

Nor set down aught in malice: then you must speak

Of one that loved not wisely, but too well;

(Othello, Act V, Sc. 2, 11. 350–352).

Introduction

In the last chapter I attempted to show how ethical meaning is involved in spirituality right from the word go. It is spirituality that provides a framework through which the ethical reflection can occur. However, it should have been clear from my explanation that this was no easy process. Inevitably a wrestling occurs, precisely because it involves testing not simply ideas but also feeling, experience and identity. This suggests that in working through any ethical issue, such as the ones noted in the last chapter, it is important, (if time allows) to enable reflection on the spiritual dimension. Spirituality in one sense underlies any relationship, in terms of particular beliefs and values. It is also evident in the somatic dimension of the relationship – how one attends to the other, how one responds creatively to the other.

In this chapter I want to look behind this process and ask what it is that actually enables it, and at the same time holds together spirituality, ethics and care. I will argue that this is love – especially the unconditional love summed up in the Judeo-Christian concept of *agape*. It is this that sustains and enables care, is at the base of spiritual awareness and provides the content for ethics. However, this view of unconditional love is not unique to the Judeo-Christian tradition, and I hope to show, similar ideas are shared by non-religious writers, such as Bauman. I will introduce my ideas in this chapter through a case study about someone who suffers a heart attack. This is not on the face of it an 'ethical problem'. However, the sense that is made of the heart attack, at various points, is suffused with values. These directly affect decisions that are made about how that person's life might change, and the subsequent ethical priorities and ethical identity of the recovering patient. In this case study we see how the development of critical moral awareness can be central to the recovery itself.

Case Study: Brian's heart attack

Early one morning Brian felt a pain in his chest, accompanied by a cold sweat. It felt quite severe but he did not want to wake his wife up or ask for help. This reflected Brian's strong moral perspective, which also meant initially he was not truly aware of the severity of this experience. Even when he began to realize the situation was very serious he refused to believe it. It was only as he went into the hospital that he begin to accept and let go of his denial. What prevented him from accepting the truth was his deep-rooted beliefs about his role and responsibility as husband. He saw himself as being the key provider for his wife. This led him to believe two things: first, that his wife would find it difficult to survive without him, and second that his wife would not longer love or accept him if he was ill. He would no longer be of any worth to his wife and thus to himself. Underlying this were Brian's principles of self-reliance and care for others, with the family as central to life.

However, alongside this awareness of his role Brian had little awareness of his physical condition. He saw himself as strong, but was not fully aware that he was three stones over weight, and that his food intake was affecting his arteries.

Brian responded with a mixture of fear and resignation to his care, and yet still harboured the hope that he might get back to life as it had been. At the end of a week he was beginning to focus more, when his wife came in to tell him that she had had a letter from the building society to say the mortgage had been paid off. When she had left, Brian broke done in tears. On seeing this the nurse assumed these were tears of joy. 'No, pet,' was Brain's response, 'I've lost the only purpose I had – that is what I lived for, to pay that mortgage.'

Brian's recovery was to involve not just a change of lifestyle but also a change of purpose and a change in his relationship to his wife and family.

In his research on victims of miocardial infarction (MI), Johnson (1991) noted several stages in the illness: onset and defence of the self; meaninglessness and chaos; finding meaning; learning to live; and living again.

Onset and defence of the self

The initial phase of a heart attack often involves denial and the attempt to defend the self. At one level this is simply about fear. The symptoms are normalized as flu or a pulled chest muscle. Some patients report checking out MI symptoms in medical literature precisely to prove 'normalcy' and many persist in this view even when symptoms become severe. At another level this involves the patient trying to hang on to their usual life-meaning. There is a concern for retaining personal control, and behind this is often the sense of a fear and even disgust of the dependency that heart trouble might bring. One patient who realized the possibility of a heart attack spoke of his fear of becoming 'a cripple'. This, in turn, affected the life-meaning attached to his family network. It was his role to maintain them and if he wasn't there then many aspects of family life would be affected, not least his daughter going to college.

Meaninglessness and chaos

The onset of illness is often characterized by a period of meaninglessness and chaos, involved in a separation from those established and core elements that offer constancy, meaning, continuance and a sense of the future.

Finding meaning

Once the truth of the condition is revealed then the patient can begin to make sense of the situation. At one level this involves facing limitations, the ultimate one being mortality. Most have some sense of unfairness, but even the question 'Why me?' is looking for some meaning. For many heart-attack victims there are also feelings of guilt. MI is often perceived as a lifestyle illness. For others there is anger that their good lifestyle has not been rewarded with health. Guilt and anger both begin to move out to the patient's network as he or she reflects on how this condition might affect life-meaning, including roles at home and at work. Will he be able to be a good parent and partner? How will this affect their sex life? How will this affect work? 'Can I really face going back to the stress and spirit-sapping conditions of work?' 'Will it mean that I cannot care for my family, provide their security?' Others experience a deeper guilt, located in a profound sense of personal shame and worthlessness. The illness can be seen as a punishment not just for their lifestyle but for the kind of person he or she is. At this point the lack of faith in the self can be cruelly exposed. For many the experience exposes a conditional ethic such as Brian's, where self-worth is dependent on role, capacity and achievement. Enabling recovery often means finding a less conditional value base.

Learning to live

Johnson suggests that for the MI victim this process involves three stages:

PRESERVING THE SELF

This is the struggle to maintain a personal identity that is not simply that of patient or invalid. In this, the patient has to reflect on and build up his or her centre of worth through reflection on their relational network. For Brian this meant working through his role and underlying belief and value systems. He also had to find a purpose that he felt gave him significance. For him, this meant moving beyond the family and looking at needs of others that he might address.

BALANCING NEEDS AND SUPPORTS.

This involves both identifying needs and negotiating appropriate support. Brian had to begin to renegotiate his relationship with his wife. In the first stages of his recovery she felt unable to give him the freedom to work through his life possibilities, and tried to do everything for him. This then led to a reassessment of the relationship. The basis for this change was both an increased awareness and acceptance of the human body with its limitations and needs, and an increased awareness of significant others, not least in the ways they give meaning to the life of the patient. Johnson talks of one MI patient who had never really perceived his wife as being separate from him. His role as provider was key to his life-meaning and once this role was questioned he found that he had not only to reassess this basis of his worth but also that he needed to begin to see his wife in very different ways – not least as someone who could operate independently of him and who could fulfil needs in ways that he had never allowed her to do before. The whole experience led to a development of mutual faith, and a sense of hope based in a relationship that was now qualitatively different no longer being simply based upon function and role, and the capacity to fulfil these. One patient reported that his wife and he had never talked so much. This led to the development of empathy that meant he could accept her fears for him and she could appreciate his desire to renew purpose and find new meaning.

MINIMIZING UNCERTAINTY

This involves the patient coming to terms with the ambiguity of the body. 'Will it let me down again?' 'Just what can I do?' 'Does recovery mean back to normal?' Such questions force the patient to focus more on the needs of their body and to develop a sense of judgement on how to respond to these. For many this was difficult. After a major shock there is generally a loss of faith in the body. Some feel betrayed by their body, others feel that they could not trust it even to the extent of not being able to sleep at night for fear of dying.

A sense of trust in the body begins to return through seeking reassurance from others, learning facts about the way the heart works, and practising cautious discernment. The process of change was seen as slow by all involved in Johnson's research and involved testing of limitations, learning to read the body and gradually modifying lifestyle. This also meant living with and accepting provisionality, the temporary or conditional nature of life.

Living again

This final stage for many is about living a new life, with greater appreciation of bodily needs and a renewed sense of purpose and hope within the context of certain limitations. These limitations may have led to changes in role and function and in some cases in a very different lifestyle. One man decided that he would retire at 55. At first sight it appeared that he was avoiding life and trying to minimize risk. In fact, he decided that work had not been a good place for him, partly because of the stress caused and partly because it had never really fulfilled him. The decision not to return was therefore a positive one that fitted into a change in the man's spiritual perception and a desire to get more from life in order to develop his sense of purpose and hope. In all this there is little sense of the person returning to 'normal'. On the contrary, some form of life-change is critically a part of the recovery.

For Brian this involved both a major review of purpose along with the renegotiation of responsibility within his family. His review of purpose, very consciously involved him in reflecting on his cultural and family background, and how his emphasis on conditional worth and value had developed. This led to him gradually sharing more responsibility with his wife, and a greater appreciation of mutual care. He did not lose a sense of conditional worth and purpose but did discover purpose that took him beyond family and to the needs of others, focused in sponsored marathon running. He developed a link to local charity, and ran for them, thus developing an involvement in a plurality of communities with related values and purposes. The running also impacted on his physical health, and had a strongly related sense of ritual, discipline and celebration (not least around his participation in the London marathon)

Critical to Brian's recovery was a move from a moral world dominated by conditional worth to a more unconditional acceptance of himself and his family. He was able to be less hard on himself, and to accept and share mutual responsibility. Along with that he began to develop a very different faith, in himself and others. The ultimate ground for this was a new awareness and appreciation of love.

Love as a basis for ethics

Some theologians argue that love can never be a coherent basis for ethics. It is simply too broad a concept. Hauerwas (1981), for example, writes that 'the ethics of love is often but a cover for what is fundamentally an assertion of ethical relativism' (p.124). The meaning of love has itself become debased in popular discourse, leading, as Hauerwas argues, to the reduction of its meaning simply to that of inclusiveness, abandoning any formerly associated ideas such as sacrifice, discipline, repentance and transformation. Hauerwas' point is that these other concepts can only be discerned through reflection on the sacrificial life of Jesus, summed up by the cross.

Such arguments suggest that there is need for care in the development of any system of ethics based on love. However, often those arguing against this provide little examination or substantive critique of the concept of love. Theologians such as Outka (1972), on the other hand, have argued that it *is* possible to develop a coherent ethics based around the concept of *agape*.

Agape
Much of the writing about *agape* has been Judeo-Christian, though the ideas are not unique to this tradition. In the Septuagint *agape* is used to translate the Hebrew *aheb*, a love centred on personal physical attraction, but extended on occasions to food or sleep (Genesis 29:18, 27:4; Proverbs 20:14). Such a love is characteristically embodied in the love of man and woman that is both physical and long term. In Hebrew there is no attempt to differentiate between erotic love based upon the attraction of the physical and the more

cooler and rational love of *agape*. Hence, even in the most erotic Song of Songs *agape* is used for love (3:1–4).

In the Old and New Testaments *agape*, not least as the love of God, is expressed in a number of vivid pictures, such as a farmer caring for his vineyard, or a shepherd for his sheep (Isaiah 5:1–7; John 10:11–16). It is a love that is even greater than a parent's love. Such a love is essentially practical, embodied, and the extent of it is summed up in John 3:16–17:

> God so loved the world that he gave his only Son, that everyone which has faith in him should not perish but have eternal life. It was not to judge the world that God sent his Son into the world, but that through him the world might be saved. (Revised English Bible, 1989)

These verses stress the inclusive aim of God's love and its nature as a gift. Indeed, the term *agape* is used in The Bible to sum up the very nature of God (1 John 4:8). Some of these ideas are summed up in William May's view (1987) of the *covenant relationships*, based on examples from the Old Testament. May argues that these relationships involve several things:

- First, it is a gift. It is not based upon any contractual terms. It precedes and may well initiate the caring relationship. In this respect the commitment is analogous to that of the family (Browning 2006). The marriage vows involve unconditional commitment. This is, if anything, intensified where there are vulnerable children needing unconditional care.

- Second, this disinterested concern for the other is one that is constant. *Agape* promises to be there whatever the response from the other. It is not simply that it is there regardless of the rights of the other. It remains true to the other whatever the other does. This is seen strongly in Hosea's image of the lover remaining faithful and calling back his lover to the relationship (Hosea 11:8–9). There are no conditions in covenant that can break that commitment.

- Third, the covenant defies precise specification and therefore remains open in terms of possibilities. It has a growing edge 'which nourishes rather than limits relationships' (May 1987). It is always searching for the good of the other.

- Fourth, the covenant is often not about an individual agreement but about one between whole communities, thus raising the possibility of an agreement that can bring many people together into a network of relationships.

May contrasts this with the 'first cousin' of the covenant, the contract. The contract is based upon conditions which, if broken, can lead to the end of the agreement. The contract attempts to sum up obligations in specific terms. This has the effect of seeing the fulfilment of the contract as discharging all responsibility. The stress in the covenant is upon the underlying relationship, and on being there for the other – any other.

This does not mean that the contract approach is wrong or unacceptable. On the contrary will be seen below it may be an important way of expressing the underlying attitude of the covenant – indeed of enabling relationships to be established and developed.

Agape in all this is both a concept and an attitude or virtue. It gives meaning but is also about existential experience. Hence, it brings together the different aspects of spirituality, ethics and care involving:

- a way of knowing and relating. As such it is the core dynamic of spirituality

- the irreducible ground of ethics, a moral attitude that precedes rational moral reflection, but also provides ethical content

- a means of empowering and motivating, and, as such, is the basis of care.

A WAY OF KNOWING

Agape has an epistemic function – that is, it is a way of revealing the other. This implies that the 'other' is not instantly accessible. Simone Weil, indeed, argues that the other is often invisible, with many factors from prejudice to fear causing this. Hence, she writes, 'If you want to become invisible, there is no surer way than to become poor'. She goes on to say, 'Love sees what is invisible' (quoted in Gaita 2000, p.xvi). Love goes beyond artificial boundaries to reveal the humanity of the other.

The dynamic of this can be expressed in the idea of empathy. Heinz Kohut characterizes empathy as follows:

1. Empathy, the recognition of the self in the other, is an indispensable tool of observation, without which vast areas of human life…remain unintelligible.

2. Empathy, the expansion of the self to include the other, constitutes a powerful psychological bond…

3. Empathy, the accepting, confirming, and understanding human echo evoked by the self, is a psychological nutriment without which life as we know it could not be sustained. (Kohut 1982, p.398)

Max Scheler (quoted in Campbell 1984, p.77) notes that is more than just fellow feeling, describing it as 'a genuine reaching out and entry into the other person and his individual situation, a true and authentic transcendence of oneself'. It is a movement beyond the concerns for the self, including fear and guilt, and with this an expansion or reaching out of the self. This involves not taking the self too seriously, and thus Scheler can write of abandoning 'personal dignity'. This is not a self-conscious process but rather one that allows the 'instinctive life to look after itself'. Such a letting go of the self is contrasted with a self-conscious concern for the other, where the concern itself begins to dominate and actually get in the way of real openness, and thus of awareness of the other. Scheler bemoans the way in which this natural awareness of the other, including the environment, has been lost, not least in a society where instrumentality – where others are used as means rather than ends – dominates.

This movement towards the other does not cause a loss of individuality to the one who cares. Indeed, the movement away from self-concern enables distance, which allows him or her to see themself more clearly. It also enhances the value of the other, enabling them to disclose what is unique about themselves to themselves and to the other. Empathy, then, is a way of knowing the other and enabling the other to know him- or herself.

There are several different key views of empathy. Two important ones come from the discipline of psychology and moral development. The first stresses the capacity to imagine how the other feels, and the stronger second one links the feelings of the other to one's own, merely identifying with those feelings. Hoffman (2000) argues that this stronger one forms the basis of caring and even justice. In effect, it is the foundation of morality. However, Kristjansson (2004) notes that neither of these meaning can act as the ultimate base of morality. He writes, 'The obvious reason for this is that the same capacity to discern or even identify with another's feelings is also a necessary condition for taking pleasure in, rather than bemoaning, the suffering for example through pure malice or *Schadenfreude*' (p.298).

Perhaps the best example of this in literature is the villain of Shakespeare's Othello, Iago. What makes Iago in one sense the ultimate villain is precisely that he understands the emotional world of all the other players so well – and, indeed, is felt by all to be a true friend who listens and counsels. This is why he is so successful at manipulating the downfall of them all. Othello himself is the total opposite. He has a great deal of love, in the sense of feeling for others, but he has little empathy. Hence, he does not fully realize the strength and character of Desdemona, and has little self-understanding, characterizing himself as 'one who loved not wisely, but too well'. So, empathy alone is not enough – it needs the moral commitment of *agape* at its base in order to see the creative possibilities in the other.

The second part of Kohut's description of empathy clearly signals this inclusive acceptance of the other and the psychological bond which this provides. Empathy is very much a working out of, and a sign of, *agape*. Without an assurance of this acceptance it would be difficult for a person to disclose anything of him- or herself. Indeed, without that love, it would be impossible to see the truth of the other. The natural human dynamic is to keep hidden that which is imagined to be unacceptable as there is always a wariness about possible judgement from the other.

Margulies (1989) has different ideas and notes four other components of empathy:

- *conceptual empathy*, stressing cognitive understanding of the other

- *self-experiential empathy*, referring to memories, affects and associations which are stirred in the listener, thus causing her to identify with the experience of the other

- *imaginative-imitative empathy*, involving imagining oneself into a model of the other's experience

- *resonant empathy*, the experience of 'affective contagion' (p.19), where the listener feels the feeling of the other (p.19).

Empathy, Marguiles argues, involves an interplay of all of these aspects, leading to an openness to the self and others and to the different as aspects of the self, whether affective, cognitive or somatic. This openness and reaching out to the other means that the empathic engagement does not deal in static truth, that is, looking behind the other to reveal *the* truth. On the contrary, if through reaching out to the other one is enabled to reveal something of oneself then the truth about the other, our awareness of the other, is continuously evolving. Facts and truth are 'a creation of the relationship itself, a continuous coming into being of possibilities requiring further exploration' (p.12).

In the light of this, empathy is both open to difference and sameness in the other. Openness to difference is characterized by wonder, surprise, curiosity and astonishment, core aspects of spirituality. Berryman (1985) notes that it is in childhood where this sense of surprise and wonder is at its height, not least because young children live at the limit of their experience most of the time. The de-centring of the self that Scheler refers to, ensures that the listener does not assert her truth on the other but is genuinely surprised by the other.

At the same time the listener comes to know the sameness in the other. Gaita (2000) notes that this is not the cognitive recognition of some generalized common humanity, but rather the recognition of what he refers to as the 'preciousness' of the other. This is a recognition that the other is one with you, a brother or sister. The startling thing is that this awareness can only be found in reaching out to the particular, to the unique other. Raymond Gaita reminds us that this sense of common bond is not a scientific universality, to do with general truth, or with abstract language, but rather the universality that we recognize in the particular, local, story of the other. Every narrator needs an 'address', needs roots, and we see our common humanity as we experience those roots, and begin to understand the roots of others in their terms and translate that story into our language. Hence:

> In literature, the universality one aspires to is of a kind that is achieved when a story or a poem in a particular natural language, historically rich and dense, shaped by and shaping the life of a people, is translated into other natural languages, historically rich and dense, and shaping the life of different peoples. (Gaita 2000, p.xxix)

In this movement, empathy involves mutuality, constant revelation of the self and other. The dynamic of this lies at the heart of genuine dialogue, dialogue that can begin to understand the other in their terms, and which can both enable and allow the challenge that comes from difference, and also enjoy the support and acceptance that comes from sameness. Sameness, involves not simply being the same as the other, but also a sense of constancy and, therefore, a sense of faithfulness. This mutual disclosure is not necessarily symmetrical. On the contrary, any relationship involves differences that lead to different aspects of the self being revealed. In the caring relationship, for instance, the carer may not reveal intimate details of her life. She will nonetheless reveal in body language and in words her attitude and her values, aspects of herself, how she feels about the other. For the person being cared for this becomes a critical narrative that she is reading from the other, as to whether she is accepted or not. For someone who comes to that relationship from a world of conditional value they are already faced with something new, and thus often hard to believe. Hence, part of the mutuality in that relationship begins to emerge through the testing of the carer's narrative. The mutuality of empathy is such that Augsberger prefers to use the word 'interpathy' (see Margulies 1989; Swinton 2001, p.141).

Empathy, then, is at the heart of awareness of the 'other', and it is precisely this that is able to hold together the different and often ambiguous aspects of the other: good/bad; same/different; particular/universal; supportive/dangerous; autonomous/part of community. Schlauch (1990) notes that this enables other tensions to be held together in knowing the other, between:

- believing and doubting. The doubting leads to the testing, and testing to a form of belief

- separated and connected (Belenky 1986). *Agape* enables the person to see the other as both different and the same

- understanding and explanation. The first involved empathic awareness, the second looks at underlying causal dynamics.

Part of Brian's recovery was precisely finding this kind of distance. He then began to see himself and his wife more clearly, and was able to initiate change and remain committed to his wife. At first he thought of his wife as a stranger, creating a prison for him. He had both to assert his needs, and understand her anxieties. At the same time he then became more aware of her needs and of how she could support him and help him change.

The ground and substance of ethics

Agape also provides a ground of ethics and for ethical content. This is focused in:

- an inclusive responsibility that transcends rules

- an ethic that exceeds a justice or rights morality

- appreciation of the particular other, and

- a mutuality that includes love of the self and that is not primarily sacrificial. Such content informs principles, rules and practice.

THE CHALLENGE OF INCLUSIVITY

Agape is a love that is unconditional, and which thus sets up an inclusivity. From a Christian perspective Schotroff (1978) reminds us that this is partly an attitude of inclusivity but that it must also lead to a concrete social event – something summed up in the command to go beyond love of neighbour to love of enemy: 'The Christian is challenged to include the persecutor in his own community... Even the enemies of the community are to be given a place in its common life and in the kingly rule of God' (p.23). This is not a make-believe world in which the enemy suddenly becomes one of us. It may be that the enemy remains the enemy, we nonetheless have to love him or her, to use moral imagination in seeing how he or she can be worked with. This sets up the extent of responsibility for the other in every situation.

Alongside this, however, is the problem that *agape* cannot be precise in ethical guidance. Indeed, Bauman (1993) suggests that there is an inescapable *aporia* in any attempt to decide what is the right course – it admits of no easy solution. The responsibility to do something about this, to respond, nonetheless, remains with the individual. Bauman contrasts the precise order or rule with the ethical demand, which is:

> abominably vague, confused and confusing, indeed barely audible. It forces the moral self to be her own interpreter, and – as with all other interpreters – remains for ever unsure about the correctness of the interpretation. However radical the interpretation one can never be fully convinced that it matched the radicality of the demand. (p.8)

Agape demands responsibility for the other and therefore some response, but at the same time we can never know if that response is absolutely right.

Faced by this demand Bauman suggests two dangers:

- First, demand can be defused by narrowing its focus. Hence, as Schrage (1988) notes, the Hebrew command to love the neighbour (Leviticus 19:18) was originally inclusive but over time was narrowed down to Israelites or full proselytes (p.73). Bauman (1993) reminds us that the key dynamic of the Holocaust was to see the Jews and others as being outside the moral claims of humanity (see also Gaita 2000).

- Second, a code of ethics can be developed. The more detailed the code, with application in many different contexts, the less the person has to take responsibility for the moral response. Indeed, the ethical rule becomes the basis of responsibility. Hence, when things go wrong there is always the plea that one was simply following the rules. However, the responsibility of love has no limits, and 'does not reach a boundary beyond which nothing is required' (Schrage 1988, p.74). This is exactly the logic behind Jesus's stress on ethical attitude in the Sermon on the Mount. The exhortation to forgive the other person seventy times seven precisely expresses a constant attitude of forgiveness, contrasted with the 'rule' of forgiving seven times, after which the person can let go of moral responsibility (Matthew 18:21–22).

BEYOND FAIRNESS

The agapeic ethic always exceeds a justice or rights morality. As Woodhead writes of the Christian perspective, its 'demands exceed legality and ask more of us than can "reasonably" be expected... The teaching of Christ is that a man does not insist even on his own rights, that he loves his enemies, that he turns the other cheek' (Woodhead 1992, p.64).

In one sense this is a love that is beyond possibility, though as Oppenheimer (1983) notes it can be embodied to some degree in human practice, not least in the example of parenting. Importantly, this means that the ethical attitude is not rational or simply calculative. Indeed, Bauman (1993) sees the starting point of morality as 'endemically and irremediably *non rational*' (p.60). Here the meaning of rationality is about survival and the capacity to calculate one's interest, something essentially defensive. Dihl goes further in arguing that the law of love is unnatural (see Schrage 1988, p.77). It is far more natural to defend one's own interest.

In this light *agape* precedes any use of rules in ethics. Woodhead (1992) contrasts this with the view of morality that is concerned 'with the regulation of the competing claims of individuals rather than with the establishment of loving personal relationships' (p.60). The first of these is achieved by 'a formal hierarchy of moral laws or rights' (p.60). The laws apply to all people and rights are possessed by all. Underlying this view is a concern for justice and fairness, and an attempt to apply ethics in a discernibly consistent, and even objective way. However, as Simone Weil (see Woodhead 1992, p.63) notes, any rights have to be founded themselves on some sense of prior obligation, and this is an obligation to the other that must be based upon need. Hence, the ethical impulse, the impulse to see the other as invaluable, precedes any attempt to calculate ends. The critical underlying point is that *agape* moves the person away from the role of spectator to direct relationship, direct awareness of the other as brother or sister, and therefore to a sense of responsibility that precedes any reflection on the particular moral response.

It would be wrong to characterize *agape* as purely non-rational. It is possible to argue rationally, with Bauman (1993), that without some point of inclusive responsibility for the other then there is the danger of looking to exclude some others. What he objects to is the use of rationality as the starting point for the ethical response, and provides ample evidence of the exclusively rational response of the Third Reich. It is also important to use rationality when working out any contract of care. This involves working through value and purpose, negotiating of responsibility, and the development of creative response – all of which require rational reflection.

APPRECIATION

Agape as unconditional love is based on the sameness of the other, and recognition and acceptance of a common humanity. Hence, Kierkegaard (1946) can write of the 'common mark' illuminated by 'the light of the eternal' (p.73). This is a love that is focused on the other, and that can thus love those who are deemed unlovable. However, *agape* also focuses on the value of the particular, in which light Tawney (1964) was able to see equality not as equal treatment for everyone but rather different treatment based on different need and capacity. Such a love is not simply about giving value to the other. Oppenheimer (1983) argues that it is also aware of and appreciates the character and quality of the other: 'It is a kind of love which looks at what people see in themselves, that positively elicits their own special character and then is glad of it: a love that creates enjoyment and enjoys creation' (p.120).

This is love, then, which is both unconditional but also involves some conditionality. Love built on the condition of attraction has often been referred to as 'eros'. Theologians such as Nygren (1932) have then set eros against *agape*, seeing eros as being purely about gratification. Love, it is argued, should be about self-giving, not about gratification. However, I would argue that polarizing the conditional and unconditional in this way runs the danger of not allowing a proper appreciation of the other.

Avis (1989) argues that the consequence of this is a disastrous dualism between the spiritual and the material. He points out that much of Nygren's interpretation of the Platonic and neo-Platonic view of love – something important to his negative view of eros – was flawed. Plato's view of eros is creative and overflowing, concerned both to give and receive. Plotinus also saw eros as a creative act, writing of its unitive role in the 'ultimate union of soul with the One' (quoted in Avis 1989, p.132). When this positive view of love is applied to a relationship with God it is found in both the energy that drives the person towards God and in the experience of the presence of God. The first of these involves transcendence of the self, not unlike the empathy described by Scheler. The second focuses on the religious experience – the sense of ecstasy at being at one with the Other (Avis 1989).

MUTUALITY

The idea of a 'one-way' love flies in the face of the Christian perspective of God's love. As Oppenheimer (1983) notes, we love God because he loves us. God loves us and desires a response, hence the making of covenant and the building up of trust. The very dynamic of empathy, as noted above, assumes mutuality not least because just as empathy enables the other to disclose herself, at the same time it involves a disclosure of the one who offers empathy. Oppenheimer (1983) refers to this as the give and take that is part of loving relationships and which is exemplified in the Trinity and the mutual caring of each person. 'God', as Fiddes (2000) puts it, 'is receptive, seeking and delighting in our response' (p.213). There has always been difficulty in this idea for some in that it implies a need on God's part. However, as Vincent Brummer (1993, p.85) notes, if we can find a part for 'need love' in healthy relationships there is no ground for seeing such need as unacceptable or bad, and no reason why we should not find an analogy in God.

SELF LOVE

As noted in the last chapter, there is a real sense in which we can see the self as an other. To exclude the self from the love of the self would therefore be inequitable. As Oppenheimer (1983) puts it:

> If any creature is to be loved and cherished, then sooner or later we ourselves are likewise to be loved and cherished…To shut our eyes to this forever would be inverted pride or faithlessness rather than Christian humility. (p.103)

The point is that such love is both unconditional, remaining committed to the self, and conditional in the sense of recognizing particular worth of the self. The balanced love that is given to the self by an other, precisely enables the person to treat his or her self in the same way. Hence, Jackson (2003) can write of a 'proper self love' (p.11) that emerges through self-transcendence.

Importantly, self love that is both inclusive and also conditional provides the moral basis for the self-critique at the heart of the ethical process. It invites the person both to accept that he or she is intrinsically of worth, and also invites them to consider their worth in practice, in what they create and how they relate. This is no cosy love, but one that sets up a tension between the self as experienced by the self and the self in relationship and response. It calls forth a response that has to reflect on purpose, practice and the relational context of both, and it gives value to and recognizes value in all of this. Hence, at the heart of *agape* is challenge.

In this there is a direct relationship between self-worth and moral meaning, and the capacity to develop moral meaning for oneself. A sense of worth based purely on conditions – be they rules, attractions or community expectations – will tend lead to a focus on the conditions of moral meaning rather than the relationships in which they are involved – that is, the humanity of the other. On the other hand, self-worth that is based purely on unconditionality, which does not challenge the person to respond (and in particular to contribute to community, thus confirming worth in action) can easily move into non-reflective self-esteem. As Richard Erikson (1987) notes, the global goal of enhancing self-esteem 'on the assumption that happiness, success and responsible behaviour will automatically follow' leads to a confused ethic that does not begin to engage with the challenges and demands of the relational network (p.163).

In the light of this it is perfectly possible to speak of a love that both desires the other and the self for their uniqueness and also loves them without condition. Jungel (1983) can thus write of *agape* as 'a power which integrates eros' (p.320).

SACRIFICE

The characterization of love as simply or primarliy other oriented also tends to stress the sacrificial elements of love, the love that will inevitably involve suffering. Feminists note the way in which such a view can easily lead to oppression. The woman is given the role of carer. Caring is seen as sacrificial. The ethical framework of this imposes guilt on the woman who tries to break out of such sacrifice and look to fulfilment beyond the family. It is hard, however, to not see some connection between suffering, sacrifice and *agape*. The very unlimited and inclusive nature of the concern inevitably means that there will be suffering in trying to achieve that. The dynamic of empathy itself is sacrificial, in the sense of reaching out beyond the self and beyond the concerns of the self. However, as Browning (2006) notes, sacrifice is not the goal of this love. Moreover, too great a stress on suffering and sacrifice can ignore inclusive and shared responsibility. This sense of mutual responsibility is at the heart of the two great commandments and also of the Christian doctrine of the Trinity. Jesus demands that we love God, the neighbour, and the self. All of these neighbours are interconnected. Such a shared responsibility is exemplified by the Trinity (Meeks 1989). The ultimate conclusion, then, of its ethic of mutuality is that *agape* is in essence social – embodied in community. This also works against an exclusively conditional or instrumental view of sacrifice, i.e. that sacrifice is offered in order to resolve or reconcile. The dynamic of reconciliation is primarily empathic, not instrumental.

PRINCIPLES AND RULES

Agape does, in fact, have substantive meaning that can be expressed in general principles. The stress on inclusivity, that sees the other as part of common humanity leads to the principles of *community* or *fellowship* – something that fits into the basic human need of belonging. Concern for particularity of the other leads to the principle of *freedom* and diversity. Commitment to the other naturally leads to the principle of *equality of respect*. Arising from these are a number of other principles such as participation and mutual responsibility.

These principles are not of themselves axiomatic in the sense of being commonly defined or accepted. The term 'equality', for instance, has at least 100 logically distinct meanings (Rae 1981). Hence, there is no simple meaning that all might agree upon prior to applying it. More importantly each of these general principles is informed by *agape*, and by each other. Community is not about the solidarity of a community over against others and the rest of the world but rather about an inclusiveness that opens communities to others, and which is thus outward looking and also self critical. The idea of freedom is not simply negative freedom (freedom from oppression or constraint) or positive freedom (freedom that enables), but involves freedom to learn, to develop, to take responsibility for the self and for the other.

In all this it is important to note that *agape* holds together all these, almost as a community of principles. The principles then enable a constant dialogue, questioning and clarifying each other. Such principles then remain constant, relevant to all situations, but never absolute in the sense of being applied unthinkingly to all situations. They enable a consistency of moral meaning but at the same time can only fully discover moral *in* the situation, through reflection on practice (van der Ven 1996, p.260). The history of ideas is peppered with writers who would argue for the supremacy of one of these above the others. *Agape* requires that *all* are taken into account as part of ethical decision-making.

In the light of this it becomes clear that *agape* relates directly to any moral rules. The moral content of *agape* provides the criteria to judge the understanding and use of any principle. The moral principle 'honour your parents' is a good example. The idea of honouring parents does not mean accepting all things that are said by the parent or obeying without question in all things. The meaning itself is tested in relation to the basic content of *agape*. Hence, honouring involves an acceptance by the child of the parents' freedom, respect for their point of view, the capacity to challenge, respect for their place in the family, and also concern for the development of mutuality. In practice this leads to a response to parents that will involve empathic listening, dialogue and mutual challenge that establishes purpose and meaning, and response that recognizes and enables the contribution of the parents and children. This set of criteria, far from eroding moral rules and principles actually strengthens them. It helps people to question and challenge so that all see what the demands of the parents are and what they mean, enabling an honouring that is mutual.

Given that rules are often used to oppress the other then it is important to continually test the use of moral principles. Even the finest of principles can be misused. Faithfulness in marriage, for instance, can be used to support acceptance of oppression and abuse – part of which may be to do with patriarchal oppression – part of which involves the build up of an alternative reality based upon conditional worth. Such a sense of conditional worth can then dominate perception so that abuse is not recognized as such. Even principles aimed at working against discrimination such as racism can be used in such a way that they oppress or oblige us to see the other as the same ignoring genuine differences (Williams 2000).

A way of empowering

The nature of love is to share power and not to take away from the other the responsibility for 'seeing' for themselves. Much that is done in the name of love ends up as manipulation. The lover is unable to wait and wants to see an immediate response from the other, or development in the relationship. Professional carers are very prone to this, not least because professionalism looks for evidence of successful outcome. Such a love might also involve doing things for the other and, once more, presents the danger of a patronizing love that cares for the other *in spite of* her failings (Bauman 1993). This is a love that actually retains the power of conditionality and thus of judgement. It wants to be good to the other but also wants the other to know that it is being so.

Agape on the other hand, involves a natural openness and is essentially vulnerable, partly because you have to wait and partly because you cannot know the outcome when you share that love. Hence, love takes one beyond the comfort zone into risk. W. H. Vanstone (1977) sums this up well:

> 'The power which love gives to the other is the power to determine the issue of love – its completion or frustration, its triumph or its tragedy. This is the vulnerability of authentic love – that it surrenders to the other power over its own issue, power to determine the triumph or tragedy of love'. (p.67)

The dynamic of *agape*, however, is more than simply one of loving and waiting. It involves a proactive reaching out with positive concern for the other, enabling response in terms of revelation of the self and testing of the other. It is this dynamic that enables the development of power. Psychotherapist Heinz Kohut (1982) sees this clearly when he argues that empathy itself, not technique, is the key to successful therapy. He sees two major aspects in empathy:

- a methodological function. It enables observation and reflection. In this the therapist is not simply giving the person an interpretation but enabling her to make her own

- as a 'psychological bond' and psychological nutriment', the very oxygen of the therapeutic relationship. Empathy in this enables both the acceptance of the self and also the growth of the self. Once again the critical sense of faithfulness and unconditional acceptance is at the core.

This is nothing less than the existential experience of care by those involved in the relationship, and the recognition of the meaning of that care.

Agape thus directly informs and enables care by those involved in the relationship, empowering the other through facilitating the articulation of narrative, reflection on meaning, and the embodiment of response – each of which we will now go and consider.

NARRATIVE

To begin with, *agape* provides the safe environment within which a person can begin to develop her narrative. Narration is critical to the development of the character, which, as van der Ven (1996) notes, is refigured 'in the twofold sense of uncovering its concealed dimensions and transforming its experienced dimensions' (p.358). Narration is a complex function that brings together all levels of awareness and meaning.

It enables the person to gain distance from the self, and so begin to become aware of experience, the effect of experience on the self, and the meaning and feelings which shape that experience. Freeman (1993) refers to this as a stage of 'distanciation', which achieves differentiation, 'a separation of the self from the self, such that the text of one's experience becomes the object of interpretation' (p.45). In this the self becomes both subject and object leading to the possibility of dialogue *with* the self *about* the self. Articulation of narrative in this sense is not simply a bilateral communication with the other. Yes, it is transmitted to the other, the listener, but it also involves the relationship with the self. The self can hear what is being said and often discovers something new about data, feelings or thoughts, something new about the self and the other. Hence, van der Ven (1996) speaks of the development of the 'dialogic self' (p.358), and of the self as both reader and writer. It is precisely this dynamic that can lead to surprises, and which enables clarification of the person's feelings and values.

REFLECTION

The more the story is articulated in the presence of another, the more it becomes reflective – and the more it focuses on the many different stories within that. As Bakhtin (1993, p.36) notes, these stories are filled with contradictions, creating not simply a universe but a 'pluriverse' or 'heteroverse', around significant others, wider communities, the environment and so on. This leads to many different dialogues, each with interactions that generate surprise, challenge and possibilities (van der Ven 1996). Such surprise and challenge are the result of contradictions or connections that might be made between the different narratives and often lead to anxiety on the part of the person who is being cared for. Once more the temptation is to reduce that anxiety through reassurance or an attempt to resolve the issue for the 'client'. However, as Halmos (1966) and Freeman (1993) note, it is crucial that the carer first enables herself to develop the dialogue so that the underlying dissonance can be seen and, second, enables her to face and work through the challenges. Only with the security and support of *agape* can the person begin to take responsibility for what for some is a risky process. The risk involves fear of sharing values and practice of which the carer may not approve.

Conflicts and contradictions that emerge between, or within, such narratives may be between:

- ideas/values and feelings
- attitude of the person to self and others
- differences between, values, beliefs and practice
- the view of the other and 'reality' of the other
- attitude and practice in the past and present
- care for others and care for the self. Often a person will show a strong narrative of concern for others and yet have quite a different narrative with regard to the self, seeing the self as not worthy of care.

The presence of the other then enables the person to examine the different narratives and the tensions between them, to test them, (including the reality of any perceptions of the other), and to either affirm meaning or work through to new meaning.

LIFE-MEANING

The development of life-meaning is critical to an individual's empowerment. It is connected to the development of identity and thus the development of the individual. As noted in Chapter 2, this in turn is connected to questions of self-worth and value – which depend upon both a sense of unconditional and conditional worth, (a sense of being accepted for the self and also being accepted because of the contribution of the self to the community) and a recognized purpose. Both of these can be seen as basic human needs, described by Kaufman (1980) as:

- A close interpersonal relationship which provides an environment of unconditional care. The experience of being nurtured.

- The experience of nurturing. This involves the practice of care for others and the assurance that this a task of value.

Agape addresses the need for unconditional acceptance experientially. Because it leads to reflection on the different narratives it also enables the person to see the nature and value of those relationships. It literally enables the person to develop empathic awareness of these others.

This reflection also begins to address the second need, i.e. the experience of nurturing. It looks at the needs and the claims of others in the relational network, the way in which they call the person to respond. It tests that calling, and tests out how the person might respond. Testing the calling of the other means a careful reflection on their narrative, what they are demanding and the reason for that demand. This is not an easy process, especially if the demands of the other have formed the basis of the person's identity and life-meaning. Hence, it involves working through the narrative at both affective and cognitive levels.

For Brian this involved a letting go of some of his meaning that was framed by family and culture. Hence, there was a sense of loss alongside any feeling of meaninglessness. This is precisely why it is important to have a holding environment of acceptance that allows the exploration of identity. It is in this environment that critique of the significant communities, and the values and beliefs they have inculcated, can be developed, without being seen as a critique of the self, or a threat to identity. Embodied *agape* empowers this reflection and questioning.

By doing this, *agape* is doing far more than simply allowing space for disinterested reflection. It is also does far more than providing confrontation that tests reality, or reflects back the narrative and its consequences. The full weight of *agape*'s empowering presence in its call to respond empathically, both to the other and the self, affirming the unconditional value of both, and thus developing the ultimate meaning of the relationship (McFadyen 1990).

For Brian this whole process was fraught with risk. At one level there was the risk of change, and developing new life-meaning. At another level risk framed the whole experience, the risk to his life. That very risk further developed his awareness, not least of the provisionality of life.

Such empowerment, then, is not simply about 'giving power' to the other. It is about both a sharing of power, and in some respects a taking of power. The carer recognizes the power of the other and enables her to use that power in the process of mutual testing. The context of that is that the caring relationship is already one in which power is imbalanced, in which the person is already in the role of 'failure', 'stranger', 'person in need'. Sharing of power in that context is about breaking down the barriers of those roles, and offering a respect that accepts the other as equal. In that relationship, the person can then begin to take and practise power.

Agape finally empowers the person to move from the new values to the new possibilities, the sharing of responsibility and the creating of new practice.

Transcendence

Transcendence has always been a key concept in writings on spirituality and now we can sum up how it relates to spirituality, ethics and care.

Transcendence is not about a separation from the world but rather is an engagement with it. Through *agape* and empathy, the person transcends him or herself, reaching out towards the other, and is able to clarify and reflect on the presence, thoughts and feelings of the self and other. Through relating to the other there is a capacity to transcend both rationality and emotions. The idea that one might transcend the 'world' through reaching out to the divine, (as it were, escaping from the world) seems difficult to sustain in this model. If this spirituality involves God then reaching out to Him is in itself engaging with another. When such a God also engages with the world, as in the Judeo-Christian tradition, then the dynamic reinforces engagement with reality, rather than taking one away from it. Articulation is the first moment of this transcendence, enabling distanciation and thus allowing the person to hear his or her self.

Second, the ensuing dialogue and critique enables the person to transcend the groups that have hitherto been the source of their beliefs and values and may have held these in place. Transcendence, however, does not demand a separation from the group. On the contrary, the very dynamic of *agape* is about acceptance and thus the capacity to continue belonging to the group while seeing it in its ambiguity.

Third, in those moments, the person also transcends the present. He or she becomes aware of the self as a person with a history, experiencing growth and development. As the present experience is transcended, so the idea of a future – of possibilities, not least the possibility of change – begins to develop.

Fourth, there is the transcendence of the limitations of the self, something about enabling the person to go beyond limitations. Parry (1988) suggests the centrality in ancient Greek culture and sport of *areté*. Often translated as 'virtue', its meaning is actually closer to 'being the best you can be', or 'reaching your highest human potential.' Of course, if spirituality is about awareness of the self and others this includes some limitations. Such awareness, however, is partly developed through testing those limitations in striving for the best. Transcendence of limitations can also be achieved through acceptance of shared responsibility, the negotiation of responsibility and the development of creative partnerships.

Finally, there is transcendence through transformation – through finding new meaning, new purpose and new practice and partnership. This is the transcendence of creative imagination and response.

Conclusion

In this chapter I have looked at the way in which *agape* holds together spirituality, ethics and care. It does so because of its inclusive commitment to the other, enabling the ethical framework outlined in the last chapter to be sustained through the development of: awareness; responsibility for the other; significant meaning; the negotiation of responsibility; and the creative response.

This is not an easy ethics, precisely because the call to love can never be fully realized, and therefore involves a continual learning process. But if that is the case, you might ask, how can it be the basis for the ethics of care professionals? It is to the ethical identity of the professions that I will now turn in the next chapter.

5

The Community of Care: Fit for Purpose

> I have been a social worker for ten years, and this is the first time I have sat down and thought about my purpose and whether I really make a difference.
>
> *(A participant in a conference on social work and ethics*
> *held at Leeds Metropolitan University 2006)*

Introduction

'The most evident bridge between morality and religion' writes Murdoch (1972, p.481) 'is the idea of virtue'. This looks to a goodness beyond fulfilling duty – one that connects ethical vision and practice. This ethics focuses on the development of character and the community of practice that embodies the core virtues. In this chapter I will look at the virtues in the context of the community of care. The chapter begins with a case study that raises questions about the nature of care in an emergency in the most difficult environment imaginable – that of Mount Everest. Using this case study, I will suggest that ethos and virtue are key to the development of spirituality and ethics, and that this can be viewed in terms of a covenantal relationship worked out through the development of contract. I then review the virtues of the caring professions and community.

On 24 September 2006 in the Sunday Times Peter Gillman reported the story of David Sharp who died on Mt. Everest in May that year.

The case of David Sharp

In May 2006 David Sharp, a 34-year-old British climber, died on Mt. Everest, from cold, exhaustion and lack of oxygen. It is thought that he had successfully reached the summit, and had then experienced problems coming down. It was Sharp's third attempt. His first, in 2003, had cost him several toes, due to frostbite, and after his second he vowed never to return. However, the lure of this astonishing mountain was too great.

Baldly stated Sharp died alone. It perhaps surprising in the first place that he should have chosen to attempt the ascent without a Sherpa. This as a man who was a trained scientist, well-known for his practical and careful thought, and who had more than sufficient funds to hire a Sherpa.

In point of fact, Sharp did not die quite alone. On the contrary his dying was in the context of a community of climbers. The broader community were those who saw themselves as responsible for the sport of climbing, those who enabled even the most unlikely to ascend Everest, such that it became part of an adventure tourist industry, those who shared Sharp's passion, and those, numbering over 200, who had died on Everest. On the day of Sharp's death this community was scaled down to some forty climbers who were aiming for the summit. Some ascending and some descending, all passed within feet of the prostrate Sharp. Many spoke in great detail of initial attempts to get Sharp to his feet, of the awful deformity caused by frostbite and of their own trauma in facing this. All moved on, up or down, leaving Sharp to his fate, and leaving the rest of the world to question what it all meant. Why did they walk by? Was there a climbing code that all were aware of and to which they adhered? Wasn't there another option? (Gillman 2006)

The story of David Sharp takes the idea of a community of care beyond the context of public services to an emergency faced by a community in which risk is very much part of its members' lives. It is a story many who read it found shocking, not least because there was amongst many climbers a view that there was a settled ethos in their community.

Spirituality and ethics come together perhaps most strongly in the idea of ethos. An ethos can be summed up as the distinctive character, spirit and attitudes of a particular group or community. As such, it is concerned with the distinctive values and meaning of that community, but also with the actual practice of those values. Thus it is summed up not just in concepts but also in how people behave towards each other, including the tone of their communication. Their ethos is discovered in relationship; in attention given, or not given, to the other; in concern for key values and purposes in practice; and in the practice itself. It could equally be referred to as the spirit or character of a community or organization.

For climbers the ethos is one that is worked out around an environment of risk shared by all. At its centre is the belief that however good any climber might be he or she might at any time have to depend upon other climbers in order to survive. Coming from that awareness of physical vulnerability, danger and need was the core principle that one always helped another climber in need. Ethicists such as McIntyre (1999) argue that concern for the other arises from an awareness of vulnerability. Such is the strength of this ethos for the climbing community that figures such as Edmund Hilary immediately condemned what they saw as its erosion in the Sharp case.

In this instance three things seemed to threaten this ethos. The first was the quest for excellence and achievement. Why was Sharp so determined to make it by himself and with limited resources? There was something about the need to prove to himself that he could do it. The irony was that Sharp had more than enough money on him to have paid for a Sherpa to accompany him. That same concern for getting to the top, come what may, was there for one man who passed him by – Mark Inglis, a remarkable New Zealand climber with two artificial legs. Inglis had himself suffered in climbing accidents and seems to have been driven by his desire to overcome his handicap.

Second, there was the seeming lack of care shown by the other climbers. The people who walked past did not even do so 'on the other side'. They had to unclip themselves from the safety line to get round Sharp. There seemed to be little awareness of any ethos and no sense of responsibility for any ethos of for anyone in need.

The third challenge to the ethos was from the commercial operation. Everest increasingly represents significant financial opportunities, with companies providing Sherpa support, and even fixed safety lines most of way up. The argument runs that this focuses the concern of the company on the profits, and purely for the care of their particular clients, ignoring the wider ethos of inclusive care for fellow climbers.

The Sharp case was complex, and many of the details are disputed. It is argued by some, for instance, that the company who had climbers on Everest that day did know of the Sharp situation and although they had the capacity to effect a rescue did not do so. Others argue the effect of extreme heights, including exhaustion and lack of oxygen, makes it very difficult to think through ethical challenges. However, it is precisely the point of an ethos that it should enable ethical response without the need to think.

In the context of professional care having an ethos is of central importance. It is difficult to see how care, in any of its corporate manifestations, can be value free. Any corporate activity expresses value, and tells us something about what that group or community find important. In the case of care, that ethos will be connected to the core purpose of caring and healing and the conditions that enable this. However, equally, the *telos* (purpose) of any organization is always contested, and depends upon perspective. I will now look at the ethos of the caring community, first from the identity and perspective of the caring professions, focusing (as an illustration) on the example of the nursing profession. Then I will look at the virtues of professional care, and finally I will consider how these translate into an ethos.

The professions

Each registered nurse, midwife and health visitor shall act, at all times, in such manner as to:

- safeguard and promote the interests of individual patients and clients;
- serve the interests of society;
- justify public trust and confidence and
- uphold and enhance the good standing and reputation of the professions.

As a registered nurse midwife or health visitor, you are personally accountable for your practice.

(The opening of the United Kingdom Central Council for Nursing, Midwifery and Health Visiting Code of Professional Conduct, 1992)

In the opening of the UKCC code, from which we have just quoted, is found a framework within which the spirituality of the profession can be explored. This preamble sets the tone and focus of the whole code. First, it implies the health-care professional is primarily there in the interest of others. None of this is to discount the interest of the professional himself – not least in earning money for himself and any dependants. Nonetheless, the underlying *raison d'être* is to serve. (The idea and wider use of the principle of service has, rightly, received some severe blows from the feminist movement. Nonetheless, although I acknowledge that the principle of service can be misused, this principle is not, *per se*, bad and can be balanced out with mutual concern.)

Second, those who the professional serves or who the profession relates to are clearly set out: the client or patient: the wider society, and the profession itself. The professional, then, is not relating to society as an individual but rather as a member of a profession whose values and identity he or she shares. Hence, how the professional relates to others affects not just his or her own relationship with the client but also the relationship of the whole profession to its members and the wider society. The profession relies upon its members to maintain the essential bond of trust with society, something based in turn on the *integrity* of the profession. Other professions, in fact, use that exact word. The American Accreditation Board for Engineering and Technology code, for instance, states that 'Engineers should advance the integrity, honor and dignity of the profession' (see Robinson and Dixon 1997, p.339). Each of these are qualities or characteristics that are required of individual practitioners, which, in turn, make up the integration, constancy, commitment, belief and value systems of the whole professional – all asserting the service-driven nature of the profession.

The identity, and thus the purpose, of professional nurses is about how they respond to the different relationships they are involved in. In turn, this sets out the plurality of their professional responsibility – to self, profession, client, broader-care community, care corporation and so on. These responsibilities require an awareness of the different needs, and the capacity to respond to the claims and call, of the different groups. Hence, the professional is not at the service of just one of those groups – is not simply an employee who has to do what he or she is told. These professionals have to determine how their service will be worked out in every different situation. Like other professions, they have a certain independence on the ground, within constraints such as safety, to work out the best way to respond in each situation they encounter.

In the later sections of the UKCC code detail is given as to what the relationships might involve in practice, spelling out:

- certain key principles such as respect, safety and beneficence

- the limitations and constraints to relating to the other

- instrumental principles, such as confidentiality

- ways of resolving conflicts, including whistle-blowing. This is more than simply an ethical dilemma, but something that is important for the integrity of the whole profession, stressing the importance of transparency

- continual development. Intellectual development is stressed along with the lengthy period of training

- basic needs of the client, including the spiritual – holistic concern for the patient.

Historically, the identity often projected onto nurses (seen as exclusively female) has been one of two extremes: the angel, the nurse as de-sexed, the ultimate carer (Campbell 1984, Ch. 3), and, at the other extreme, the technician whose task it is to save lives. The first is all care, the second is all competence. Neither is human and neither reflects the complex and rich spirituality of nursing care that holds together both care and competence. I would argue that this combination is held together in the concepts of covenant and contract.

Covenant and contract

The spirituality of the caring professions tends to be based upon covenant rather than contract. As noted in Chapter 4, May (1987) sees the covenant as embodying unconditional care. It is:

- *Gift-based.* The caring professions offer care to society based upon need, not upon ability to pay. Titmuss (1970) takes this further with the concept of caring for strangers, an inclusive/unconditional offer. In this sense the action of care can be seen as sacramental – as a sign that points to a broader view of care, taken beyond simply individual response. The health service as a whole can be viewed as a sacrament of care.

- *Promissary.* The profession remains available whatever the response of the patient or client. If need arises beyond the contacted hours then there is a duty to respond.

- *Open.* The commitment of the caring professions defies precise specification. In this sense the precise responsibility of the profession can only be worked out in the particular situation through further dialogue. This can be contrasted with the more exclusive view that professions have their responsibility predetermined. This openness to the situation enables space for creative response.

- *Community-based.* The profession forms part of a wider community and group of communities that share interlocking aims, and which work together to achieve those. For all its problems in delivery, the National Health Service is a good example of this.

By the side of the covenant of care is the idea of contract. A contract is specific, calculative and limits relationships, and can be put to one side if the terms of the agreement are broken. It would be very easy to polarize these two approaches to agreements and lead to a battle between covenant and contract. Titmuss (1970), for instance, saw the two as mutually exclusive foundations to any national health service and advocated the gift relationship based upon 'ultra obligations' (p.240) – obligations that were more than simply family or tribal ties. Hence, for him the contribution to any health service had to be anonymous – genuine stranger giving, as in blood-donorship.

However, important though this theme is to the profession, it runs the danger of obscuring the important part that contract can play in professional spirituality. The covenant emphasizes the unconditional 'being there', and the attempt to be aware of the network of different relationships involved in the caring relationship. The contract emphasizes the specific activity and outcome of the healing relationship, and thus stresses a spirituality of 'doing'. A contract enables expectations to be clear and boundaries drawn – so that the professional remains in role. This also enables clear expectations for the patient or client. The limitations of care can also be focused on, and, therefore, the best stewardship of those resources. In focusing on the specific, the contract can also focus on the professional competence – the capacity to maintain standards of care.

Any spirituality of the profession needs both of these elements. Nonetheless, there is an importance in basing the contract in a covenant framework. First, it is always possible to move from the unconditional to the specific, but very difficult to move the other way. Second, the contract is necessary if the unconditional and inclusive care is to become a reality. The two, in fact, involve the twin axes of spirituality – sameness (care that is based upon the recognition of common humanity), and difference (care which takes account of the particularity of a person and of her situation and need). Of course, the openness of the covenant will never be fully 'achieved' but that is not a reason for not continuously working towards it.

PROFESSIONALISM

It would, however, be wrong to ignore the ambiguity that lies at the heart of any profession. George Bernard Shaw summed up the popular image of the professions as 'conspiracies against the laity' (*The Doctor's Dilemma, act 1.*) concerned primarily for their own interests. At the bottom of this is the danger of defending the profession and keeping power to itself, something not completely unknown in the development of the NHS (Baggott 1994), and which, in turn, can lead to a resistance to change.

A second danger is that of professionalization. This stresses the exclusive skills and status of members of a profession. Moreover, it tends to see such skills as unique and as not to be practised by those outside the profession. In one sense this is reasonable. In another it has the danger of creating a polarization that does not value the contribution of others to the health process, neglecting the wider community's health-care resources. Stress on the expertise of the health-care worker can easily lead to a stress on power and to the diminishment of the patient, encouraging dependency and infantilization (Campbell 1984).

A third danger suggested by the history of professionalization is an increased stress on the intellect. This often goes hand in hand with stress on scientific methods. Not only can this lead to the loss of the development of crucial holistic skills, it also can lead to a scientism that both sees the patient as a case and also relies more and more on scientific techniques for diagnosis, rather than more relational holistic judgement.

Professional virtues

The word 'virtue' comes from the Latin *virtus* which is stems from *vir*, man. *Virtus* means 'the male function' expressed in terms of strength or the capacity to accomplish. In this sense, virtues are the qualities of the person that enable something to be brought into being, i.e. moral virtues enable moral meaning and purpose to be embodied. By extension they are the qualities that enable a spiritual ethos to be lived out in individual and corporate practice. Hence, we would normally refer to the virtues of the individual, but it is also possible to use the term in relation to a community or group – i.e. describing a group as having integrity.

Professional codes of practice aim to set out ethical expectations. However, they can also begin to set out a framework for spirituality. Codes and processes can be useful in reminding the professional of important relationships and of the ways in which they should be approached. However, codes and processes in themselves can never be a substitute for spiritual awareness and attitudes of care because by their very nature, they tend towards generality whereas spirituality focuses also on the particularity of the other. Reliance upon codes has the danger of taking away from the professional the responsibility for responding to the other. No code should be operated without judgement and awareness. Codes should focus on the virtues and skills of the carer, enabling both caring presence and also the humane use of technique. Technical competence thus becomes part of caring.

One way of setting out virtues is through a taxonomy of qualities and skills, such as that set out by Richard Carter for professional education in general (Carter 1985) in Table 5.1.

The taxonomy sets out the different qualities, skills and knowledge and suggests that they relate to each other. Attitudes and values involve virtues, such as respect for the self and others and integrity, and spiritual qualities including awareness. Such virtues relate directly to skills. Information skills, for instance operate in the context of respect, and remembering and communication can themselves express respect and care. The virtues of openness and imagination tie in directly to good organizational and planning skills. Indeed, creativity is precisely expressed in such skills. Without them it would not be clear what creative imagination was. As McIntyre (1981) notes, virtues are internal to skills, and the virtues are developed through practice of the skills.

Table 5.1. A summary of a taxonomy of objectives for professional education (Carter 1985)

Personal qualities	Mental characteristics	Attitudes and values	Personality characteristics	Spiritual characteristics
	Openness	To Things	Integrity	Awareness
	Agility	Self	Initiative	Appreciation
	Imagination	People	Industry	Response
	Creativity	Groups	Emotional resilience	
		Ideas		
Skills	Mental skills	Information skills	Action skills	Social skills
	Organization	Acquisition	Manual	Cooperation
	Analysis	Recording	Organizing	Leadership
	Evaluation	Remembering	Decision-making	Negotiation and persuasion
	Synthesis	Communication	Problem-solving	Interviewing
Knowledge	Factual knowledge		Experiential knowledge	
	Facts		Experience	
	Procedures		Internalization	
	Principles		Generalization	
	Structures		Abstraction	
	Concepts			

Yorke and Knight (2004) suggest a four components view of employability that precisely links deeper meaning to competence:

- *Understanding.* This is intentionally differentiated from knowledge, signifying a deeper awareness of data and its contextual meaning.

- *Skills.* This refers to skills in context and practice and therefore implies the capacity to use skills in the context of professional values.

- *Efficacy beliefs, self theories and personal qualities.* These influence how the person will perform in work. There is some evidence, for instance, to point to malleable, as distinct from fixed, beliefs about the self being connected to a capacity to see tasks as learning opportunities rather than opportunities to demonstrate competence (p.5). This, in turn, influences commitment to learning goals and the capacity to learn.

- *Metacognition.* This involves self-awareness, and the capacity to learn through reflective practice.

The first of these can involve both doctrinal and affective meaning. The second sets skills in their context of meaning. The third involves identity. The final category is precisely the reflective capacity that enables self-transcendence and with that the ability to see how one thinks, feels (in relation to thought) and learns.

I would suggest that there are four virtues that are particularly important for the professional carer: practical wisdom; empathy; integrity and *agape*.

PRACTICAL WISDOM

This is Aristotle's virtue of 'phronesis', the capacity for rational deliberation, that enables the wise person to reflect on her conception of the good and to connect this to practice. Aristotle sees this not as a moral virtue but as an intellectual virtue. At its core is reflection on purpose (Aristotle's *telos*). Sternberg (2000) contrasts this with teleopathy – choosing and following a purpose that is against or not to do with the profession. Clearly, professionalization as described earlier is teleopathic. Equally, well-intentioned practice such as targets, be they quotas or cutting down waiting times, can become teleopathic. This is most obvious in practice that focuses on task fulfillment rather than relating to the patient or client, on techniques rather than tone. Phronesis then is not a precious virtue, to be confined to philosophical discourse. Rather, it is at the heart of everyday care planning and relationships. In both areas the practitioner needs to ask that question, 'Am I remaining true to purpose'. Only in the light of that can we assess what 'fitness for purpose' is.

Practical wisdom for Aquinas (1981, IIaIIae 47.6) had at its heart three elements: openness to the past (*memoria*), openness to the present (involving the capacity to be still and listen actively (*docilitas*)) and openness to the future (*solertia*). This stresses openness and care before making any hasty judgement or decision. In being open to the present and the future this wisdom also stresses an appreciation of reality and thus of both constraints and possibilities in any situation. Because of its concern for reality, Aquinas saw this type of wisdom as being at the foundation of the virtues. It is also one that works against a simple utilitarian view of wisdom – and thus against a primarily target-centred approach to professionalism. As noted above, targets can become a substitute for responsibility and take the focus away from person-centred care.

Campbell (1984) suggests three ways in which practical wisdom is developed in the context of care:

- Wisdom as *folly*, reaches out to the patient in her vulnerability, the opposite of simply technical wisdom which simply looks to reduce risk.

- Wisdom as *simplicity*. This starts from direct personal engagement rather than from the increased technical sophistication of medical technology.

- Wisdom as *discretion* – knowing when to intervene and when to remain silent. This is often thought of as an intuitive skill. However, it is, rather, a function of the openness referred to above. The idea of intuitive knowledge is itself often either sketchy or romanticized, coming as if from nowhere. It is better to see it as a spiritual quality that is making the best use of affective, cognitive and somatic knowledge.

Phronesis is a virtue necessary both to maintaining the identity of the carer, and therefore also their competence, because it focuses on the underlying meaning and experience of care.

EMPATHY

Empathy is closely connected to the virtue of benevolence, and enables the professional to identify with the other. If wisdom is an intellectual virtue then empathy is an affective virtue. It is the capacity to hear and understand underlying feelings. This involves an awareness of others and their needs, regardless of who they are, or whether they are a member of the community (cf. McIntyre 1999, p.122ff. on the virtue of *misericordia*).

Empathy does not mean total identification with someone (sympathy), but rather enables an appropriate distance between the self and the other. Such a distance is necessary if the other is to be understood, and if the professional is to operate impartially and effectively (Robinson 2001). As such, empathy forms the basis of the professional carer's perception, data collection and judgement, including the skills of diagnosis. Similarly, empathy enables the professional to be aware of and accept his or her own limitations, and to avoid the kind of self-conscious caring that wants to impose their own needs on the relationship.

As I noted in Chapter 4, the dynamic of empathy is one of mutuality. Mayer notes the lack of attention to this dynamic in the caring community (Mayer 1992), 'Care is seen as something delivered to the powerless from the powerful. There is little awareness in the literature of the patient's capacity to give and thus create a mutual relationship' (p.52). Campbell notes the mutual grace of such a relationship, and how the response from the patient can often enable the care of the nurse (Campbell 1984, see also Griffin 1983):

> The professional, who is aware of how much he or she gains in support, enlightenment and personal development from helping others, may well feel a greater indebtedness. It is often more blessed to care than to be cared for: and the ability to care is frequently made possible by the understanding and sensitivity of the needy person. Such reciprocity suffuses the relationship of caring with a spontaneity, with a sense of grace which enriches carer and cared-for alike. (p.107)

Such an empathy also enables an awareness of colleagues in associated professions, and of the limitations and vulnerability of the carer themselves (Nouwen 1994).

It is worth underlining, however, that whilst empathy is a key virtue that caring professionals need to develop in order to fulfil their purpose it is not exclusive to these professions, and thus can't be claimed specifically as a counselling or nursing skill. Empathy, as I suggested in Chapter 4, is a foundation of spiritual awareness. As such it is a human quality, a 'transferable' virtue. Such a human quality, of course, has to be used with great intentionality in certain areas of human practice, including counselling. It is also necessary for effective diagnosis, for wider pastoral care, and for effective management and so on.

Several skills, such as listening and communication skills, are based in empathy, all of which demand an attitude of openness. It is easy, especially in professional training, to focus on the skills, seeing them as a form of technique and thus not seeing them as related to, or based, *in*, the self, or in the context of the community and its values.

Empathy and practical wisdom both connect the concern of ethics with professional competence. Both enable appreciation and care of the other and both support imagination, and openness, key to the creative process and making effective decisions. Qualities such as imagination can also affect awareness of the other, and thus the development of empathy. Such virtues and capacities enable holistic thinking and practice, and thus effective engagement with the ethical issues at the heart of the professions and business. Both relate directly to technical knowledge, providing the meaning structure within which that knowledge can be practised.

INTEGRITY

Solomon (1992) suggests that integrity is not one virtue but a collection of several virtues, which come together to form a coherent character and identity.

This involves, first, making connections between the different aspects of the self (cognitive, affective and somatic), and the self and practice. This then leads to holistic thinking that takes account of how the feelings, thoughts and physicality affect each other, enabling thinking that is affective and feeling that is cognitive.

Somatic awareness is equally important, not least because, as David Ford (1999) notes, all action involves communication. To put it another way, all action embodies in some way attitude and values. Somatic awareness is at the base of spirituality at the earliest stages of human development. Stern (1985) notes research on early childhood, that demonstrates the establishing of shared affect as early as nine months, including an awareness of congruence between the facial expression of another and the baby's own affective state. If the care-taker's face expresses anxiety about a new or dangerous situation the baby will also express this and turn away from the danger. Behind this lies what Stern calls 'affect atunement', a complex, dynamic and ongoing operation which involves the care-taker in recognizing the affective state of the child and communicating that recognition. It is a communication through tone and body attitude that the care taken is 'in resonance, in synchronicity' with the experience of the baby (Stern 1985, p.129). It is precisely this level of communication that is later discouraged in different ways as the child develops or which leads to contradictory messages coming from care-takers that cause the child to build up a confused and anxious life-meaning. Hence, Rogers (1983) was precisely right to stress the need for congruence in the attitude of the carer. A critical part of the caring process then becomes learning a level of awareness which had been in some way discouraged, and with that learning to trust the embodied other.

Second, integrity involves a constancy and consistency between: the self, values and practice; past, present and future; and different relationships, situations and contexts. The response may not be exactly the same in every context but will remain consistent to the identity and purpose of the person. Central to this is the idea of being true to the self and thus faithful to the self.

A third aspect of integrity is honesty or transparency. This is partly about an openness to the self and others and partly about remaining focused on the truth of a narrative. Such a truth is, of course, no simple objective truth found separate from the network of relationships. As Smail (1984), notes much of 'truth' about ourselves and others is illusional. I might see myself as different and strange, unable to cope, and unable to live up to the excellence that is evidenced in others. This, in turn, is reinforced by media images, which set up standards of adequacy that people can find hard to live up to. This then leads to people being unwilling to disclose the real anxiety and chaos that they experience, even to themselves. Honesty is thus very much about how one is able to examine oneself and others in a way that both accepts and tests one's illusions.

A fourth element in integrity is responsibility including responsibility for meaning and purpose. If someone simply accepted the meaning and purpose supplied to them by the other then there would be no separate identity, and no attempt to relate to the different aspects of experience. Therefore, an important part of integrity is the testing and developing of purpose with and in relation to others. Without accepting responsibility for ethical values and for response neither the individual nor the profession can develop a genuine moral identity or agency. This also demands independence, ensuring epistemic and functional distance, such that the professional can stand apart from competing interests, and more effectively perceive and understand the core purpose.

Given the limitations of human beings it is impossible to have complete integrity in any static sense. Integrity is best viewed in terms of a continual learning process, with the person discovering more about the different aspects of the self and others and how these connect. Central to this is the capacity to reflect, to evaluate practice, to be able to cope with criticism and to maintain, develop or alter practice appropriately. This is not a matter of someone just seeking wholeness, more a question of the person becoming more 'at one' with the self and others.

AGAPE

We have already noted the part that love (*agape*) plays in spirituality and ethics, as a way of being, knowing, learning, and empowering. It is important, however, when viewing *agape* as a professional virtue to see how it is located in the practical context. Campbell (1984) notes how it is highly practical. It generates empathy and thus is balanced – enabling professional distance as well as particular concern. It is not simply an affect but a matter of the will, enabling responsibility for meaning and practice. It does not attempt to dominate but enables the other to take up their freedom, treating them as subject not object. It recognizes and appreciates the common humanity of the other, never losing a sense of their particular needs. *Agape* is the virtue that lies at the base of the covenant attitude, with an inclusive unconditional care for the other. As such, it is very close to the unconditional positive regard used by counsellors (Rogers 1983). *Agape* enables and informs empathy and integrity. It also informs the *phronesis* (practical wisdom), precisely because *agape* informs the core purpose of care, and works against the teleopathy of care.

Agape also involves *veracity* and *fidelity*. Veracity is not simply about telling the truth to the patient (an issue about which there has been much sterile ethical debate). It is more about sharing the truth with the patient in such a way that he or she can begin to take responsibility for it. The carer in this takes on a pedagogical role enabling the patient to reflect and to explore. Genuine reflection and exploration will not only enable someone to begin to handle the truth about the self which has been reflected back by the carer, it will also explore the different possibilities for the futures – for example, in relation to an illness. Such a dialogue enables any truth about a patient's condition to emerge. Fidelity is also about truth, in this case remaining true *to*, in the sense of being committed to, the client.

As the caring contract is worked through in the therapeutic relationship so is the underlying love moderated, focused in the particular relationship, and the needs of the client (Campbell 1984).

Virtues and professional principles

Close to some of these virtues seem to be the four principles put forward by Beauchamp and Childress (1994) as the ground of medical ethics:

- respect for the autonomy of the patient
- beneficence (enabling the best for the patient)
- non maleficence (avoiding harm to the patient), and
- justice.

Armed with these Gillon (2003) argues that virtue ethics cannot by itself provide moral content to the professional. He cites the case of the 'sincere ethnic cleanser', the man who had all the Arisotelian virtues – perseverance, justice, courage and so on – but chose to use them to a bad end. Gillon wants to argue that any virtue is dependent upon the logically prior content of moral principles. The problem with this argument is that logical priority assumes that the meaning of the four principles is clear. Respect for autonomy, for instance, could mean several things, and thus is itself dependent on some other prior meaning. Justice also has many different meanings, which are in turn dependent upon the underlying view of humanity one chooses.

Campbell (2003) argues that principles such as those of Beauchamp and Childress are complementary to the virtues. Even such complementarity, however, depends on the meaning one gives to the principles. I would argue that the only effective base to principles or virtues is *agape*, because it provides both the irreducible moral attitude of inclusive care (care for all), and because of its impetus to respond to the other. Indeed, common definitions of terms such as empathy assume a context of care for the other. Building on the core virtues are several others. The four principles then become complementary in the light of their being interpreted by *agape*. Hence, justice, for instance, will focus on a wide variety of meanings, not least restorative justice, and respect will be more than simply a form of negative freedom.

Other virtues
EROS
Regarding eros as a virtue ushers in the possibility of a virtue that is gratifying, that actually enables existential pleasure for the professional. The term 'existential pleasure' was coined by Florman (1976) around the profession of engineering. Engineering, he suggests, is an attempt to engage with and utilize the social and physical environment in order to fulfil human needs, desire and aspirations. Similarly, it could be said that the caring professional attempts to engage with persons in the physical, psychological and social context in order to enable human health and well-being. This might involve several existential pleasures:

- The very act of being able to change the world in some way. There is a human impulse to change and improve, and to make a difference. This is close to Erikson's idea of generativity (1959).

- The joy of the applied scientist, who is able to begin to understand medical science and research in the context of care.

- The pleasure of service. In this the caring profession would not differ greatly from Florman (1976) who writes, 'The main existential pleasure of the engineer will always be to contribute to the well-being of his fellow man' (p.147).

There is nothing wrong with gratification gained from professional work *per se*, ranging from a feeling of well-being from a job well done to a passionate concern for research. This generates important meaning in the job as the contribution of the person and the profession can be clearly seen and appreciated. Meaning then emerges from the sense of value. Such pride can be an important motivation for maintaining competence and care. It has its religious analogue in relation in the creation. God appreciated his work and 'saw that it was good' (Genesis 1:21). This virtue also relates to *areté*, the idea of human excellence.

HUMILITY

In his Socratic dialogues, Plato identified particular virtues associated with *areté* as being piety, temperance, courage, and justice (see Reid 2006). Piety involves awareness of, or obedience to, a god, or something or someone that is greater than oneself, and actions or ritual that demonstrates this awareness. Reid (2006) suggests that this can be recast as self-knowledge or awareness. This relates closely to the virtue of humility, defined as an awareness of the limitations as well as the strengths of the self. The point about piety is that awareness of something greater than oneself puts the self into perspective, thus enabling a realistic assessment of the self. A professional's humility involves a proper appreciation and acknowledgement of the contribution of the profession and of the authority in the profession.

The virtue of *humility* is often seen as irrelevant to professions. However, in one sense it is an important corrective if the expertise of the professional becomes a *raison d'être* or the basis of status or identity. Humility is often seen as meaning a nervous doubting of competence or self deprecation – quite the opposite of the professional image. Tangney (2000), however, summarizes a very different view of humility, reminding us that all virtues rest between extremes. Humility involves:

- accurate assessment of one's ability and achievements

- ability to acknowledge one's mistakes, imperfections, gaps in knowledge and limitations

- openness to new ideas, contradictory information and advice

- keeping one's abilities and accomplishments – one's place in the world – in perspective

- relatively low self-focus, 'a forgetting of the self', while recognizing that one is but part of a larger universe

- appreciation of the value of all things, as well as the many different ways that people can contribute to our world. (p.74)

HOPE
This involves:

- The capacity to create hope, connecting closely with openness to the future.

- The capacity to make a client feel that they are not hopeless – hope here as arising out of the experience of acceptance.

- The capacity to be hopeful. Professionals themselves need to have grounds for hope, ranging from the possibilities for professional promotion to the different ways in which they can affect the healing process. Connected to that is the capacity to work creatively with colleagues and thus increase possibilities.

Underlying such virtues are other traditional virtues, associated with Aristotle and Plato (May 1994):

- *Temperance.* This does not mean abstinence – from drink or anything else, but rather moderation, balance and self control. This is important for effective judgement, self-reliance and the acceptance of responsibility. Reid (2006) suggests that Plato's *sophrosune*, (temperance or self-control) corresponds to discipline. Discipline, in the sense of keeping to training or eating regimes, is, however, only part of this virtue. It also includes a sense of balance, of not moving to extremes, and is therefore essential in the exercise of judgement.

- *Justice.* This involves both the capacity to maintain contracts (commutative justice) and the capacity to give equal regard and respect for all groups and issues in any situation. It also includes restorative justice.

- *Fortitude/courage.* This involves courage and resilience and the capacity to withstand a variety of pressures. Like all Aristole's virtues this involves the mean – in this case between the extremes of foolhardiness and cowardice. Courage for Plato is quite a complex idea. It is not about thoughtless bravery. It includes a capacity to persevere with an aim, whilst also holding a critical relationship to that aim, enabling one to modify it as and when it is right to do so. Again, there is tension in this virtue, between the courage to stick something out (literally going the extra mile, surviving perhaps great suffering) and knowing when to stop.

Clearly precise definitions of any of the virtues can vary and an important part of professional training can be to invite the student and practitioner to reflect on these and describe them in their own ways. Several things are, however, clear:

- The virtues are not simply individualistic. They are related to the whole and thus can be used and practised only in the light of the support of the wider community. Similarly, no individual could embody all the virtues. Hence, team members might embody different ones, enabling the whole team to embody all the virtues. This also means accepting the limitations of team members. One can also view a community as a whole as the bearer of virtues. Hence, we can speak, for instance of structural or group empathy.

- Virtues need to be maintained, encouraged and practised. They do not develop without such disciplines. The development of virtues is a life-long process. Hence, the concern for continual professional reflection (Schoen 1983).

- Virtues are not context specific. Nor are they the virtues of expertise. On the contrary, as we noted above, they are the virtues of humanity *per se*, which can then be applied to different contexts.

- The virtues are interrelated and inter-dependent. Hence, whilst no one person can embody all the virtues, Aristotle believed that one could not develop the virtues singly.

- The virtues are the same across the different caring professions. *Phronesis*, empathy, integrity and moderated love in particular are core to professional competence and care. Different professions will work these through in distinct intentional relationships, but they remain important to all.

Virtues are necessary for the delivery of professional care, including spiritual care and the capacity to respond ethically. On the other hand, virtues also involve the spiritual needs of the carer. Carers need a sense of unconditional acceptance, a work context that they can put their faith in and which gives the space to work through their life-meaning, the development of hope and so on. This suggests the need for another view of love – *philia*, meaning friendship or solidarity. Part of this will be provided by the learning environment and part by the ethos of the workplace itself.

Ethos

Up to this point I have looked at the identity and purpose of the professional carer in terms of both service and gratification, and the virtues that enable the purpose of care. This all assumes the existence of a community of practice and an ethos that embodies those virtues. But what would such a community look like?

First, it would be a plural community. This means an overall community of care that includes the discernible caring communities of the different professions. Each of the professions have their own statement of purpose and ethical code. These provide something of an ethos and ethical identity, framed around a particular community of practice. (In practice, however, it is easy for fragmentation to occur, and for members of that community to lose a sense of shared identity and ethos. In turn, as Bauman (1989) reminds us, this can lead to the fragmentation of responsibility and thus of service. Such fragmentation can occur partly as a function of size and partly through a lack of an ethos of shared responsibility.) Such a community can be distinguished from, but includes, the institution of care, e.g. the hospital. The institution or corporation is the entity that has the responsibility for resourcing and delivering care. Hence, it is critical that the administrative professions are part of the community, contributing towards reflection on purpose and creative response.

Second, it would be a learning community. Hawkins (1991) refers to the spiritual dimension of the learning organization. He argues that beyond the level of operations and strategy the developing organization needs to attend to questions of underlying identity and purpose. At this level there is the development of 'integrative awareness' (p.178) which ensures that there is transparency and participation such that all involved recognize shared life-meaning and begin to accept mutual responsibility and interdependence. I would add to this the need to attend to integrity. This can be achieved though good planning, which allows wide participation in reflecting on purpose, aims and objectives. Integrity can facilitate the learning process in an organization. One example of this is the provision of whistle-blowing and anti-bullying procedures that enable transparency such that conflict can be dealt with constructively (Wright and Sayre-Adams 2000). Perhaps more important is the inclusion of all members of staff, e.g. in the local practice, in developing a spiritual framework, including:

- articulating value statements and the ethos
- identifying value conflicts for the team/organization
- ensuring effective responsibility sharing and valuing of different roles
- developing creative responses to patient needs.

This would require space for staff reflection on a regular basis – reflection that itself could facilitate the development of structural empathy and *phronesis*.

Third, it would be a community that connects and transcends. Much of professional life is seen in terms of bolt-on extras – another skill to be learned, another perspective to take on board. The ethos of the caring community should be to integrate meaning with practice. Schoen's (1983) reflective practice, for instance, provides an ideal focus for the connective and learning community. It includes reflection on values and 'appreciative systems' (overarching theories that supply meaning to any situation) and the roles of the professional and others involved. Moreover, Schoen usefully refers to the 'talkback' (the articulation of the different phases of reflection) that provides the basis for adjusting future practice, and argues that the professional should treat the client as a reflective practitioner. It is easy to draw an ethos from this. The management of change is handled well through evidence-based practice (Hamer and Collinson 1999), which also ties into underlying values and beliefs. Indeed, establishing together the shared values and purpose is a key to handling change.

Connecting to wider value is exemplified by care teams who have made links with the wider care community through a sense of corporate social responsibility. One primary-care team, for instance, had a link to a primary-care team in South Africa, and placed photos and reports in the waiting room, encouraging patients to get involved in the link, contributing things such as old books, stamps, etc. The aim here was to transcend the immediate care horizon and set up reflection that would engage empathy, and make all feel an active part of a caring community. Gift-giving, as Titmuss (1970) argued, can establish rituals that reaffirm the altruistic base of the caring community. Such rituals can clearly embody basic values, and further develop integrity. Such rituals remind us that ethics is not just about ethical dilemmas. Levine (1990) writes:

> There are overlooked ethical challenges in the mundane everyday activities of professional practice and these have gone largely unexamined. Ethical behaviour is not the display of one's moral rectitude in times of crisis. It is the day-to-day expression of one's commitment to other persons and the ways in which human beings relate to one another in their daily interactions. (p.41)

Fourth, it would be a genuinely interprofessional community, in which the skills and presence of other professionals are valued in relation to the shared purpose and values. One of the most striking examples of this is the role of the 'housekeeper' on hospital wards, the impact of which was investigated by O'Neil (2006). Whilst support for the housing keeping role has not been universal (partly because of budgetry issues) the results of the survey were remarkable, as shown in the following quote from O'Neil's publication:

Patient experience

1.1 Housekeepers get to know patients and carers over time and this supports the provision of a more personalized service.

1.2 Housekeepers bring a sense or normality and homeliness to busy clinical environments. Reports of housekeepers offering comfort and reassurance to patients and family are common.

1.3 Patients value being able to develop different sorts of relationships with housekeepers than they do with clinical staff. This was particularly evident in mental health and learning disabilities settings.

1.4 First point of contact, therefore creating a positive early impression. Housekeepers in many organizations play a role in settling people into the ward, giving information to patients and relatives. This was often described as meeting a need that goes beyond the clinical/medical side of things and links in to what we know about the emotional aspects of being in hospital.

1.5 Housekeepers themselves really value being able to make a difference to patients and carers and having the opportunity to make small but significant improvements.

Linking-pin

1.6 Being the 'eyes and ears' of the ward. Housekeepers get to know patients and can often detect significant changes and also safety issues and feedback this information to the clinical staff.

1.7 Coordination and integration of clinical and non clinical aspects of care and brings Facilities and Hotel Services expertise directly into the clinical environment.

1.8 Supervision of domestic staff and reporting of issues to the ward manager.

1.9 Liaison with catering staff and influencing the type and method of food service.

Freeing nursing time

1.10 Nurses and patients report that housekeepers free up time for nurses to focus on clinical tasks. The study showed that in wards where a housekeeper is present the proportion of time given over by nursing staff to non-nursing work is about 15%. In wards where a housekeeper is not present this proportion is about 19%, a difference of 4% between the two groups. In one site, a study conducted over a year found that 18 hours a week of nursing time was saved after the introduction of a housekeeper.

(O'Neil 2006, pp.24–25)

Housekeepers in some wards had become an integral part of the caring community. They were given a voice in developing the ethos, and were valued by other colleagues and patients. Their contribution:

- affected the physical and social environment of the ward, making it more homely

- released time for other colleagues

- directly affected the patients, in that many felt more able to talk to them rather than a busy nurse or doctor

- reinforced the caring ethos of the ward, and helped to focus on purpose and meaning beyond the immediate care of the wards and the pursuit of technical expertise.

Fifth, training and development would reflect these issues, enabling the development of virtues as well as skills. Some argue that virtues cannot be taught, they are either inherited or 'caught'. Others argue that virtues are identified and developed through living in communities and through the reiteration of, and reflection on, the community stories. These stories illustrate or embody the virtues (McIntyre 1981). Indeed, such stories focusing on practice are the only way of actually understanding the virtues. They cannot be understood apart from action. Even this approach runs the danger of imposing a view of the good or a view of the spiritual. In this view the virtues are transmitted or infused, a predetermined spirituality which is passed across.

However, virtue development in the light of the spirituality noted thus far is a little different. So far we have agreed that the virtues would develop through the practice of the caring relationships and through reflection and dialogue between the many different groups that make up the caring community. This reflection would itself set up dialogue, mutual challenge, empathy and *phronesis*, as well as commitment to the other. Interprofessional training becomes important, then, for the development of a shared ethos, and not just for improving technical skills.

Sixth, the caring community would embody mutual support. This includes support for staff when their spiritual and moral meaning is challenged (Wilcock 1996). Nouwen (1994) suggests that all healers are wounded in some way. If this is true it demands an ethos and procedures that both encourage the development of high professional skills and competence but also ensure that limitations are accepted, and support is available where needed.

The ethos of the caring community, then, should embody the core virtues of *phronesis*, empathy and integrity, such that the core purpose of care is made clear in:

- mission and value statements
- the quality of attention offered
- the physical arrangement of the community.

(Department of Health and King's Fund 2006)

Such an ethos can be further enhanced by reflection, rituals and celebrations of health and care. Even functional activities of care, such as taking blood pressure, can become actions that remind patient and carer of the nature and purpose of care, not least through the carer helping the patient to understand how what is being done relates to the care. Larger celebrations include health awareness events reaching across schools, and wider communities. Such events enable a reflection on a broader view of health and care, one that stresses shared responsibility for both. Again, these can be shared across the wider community, with educational and community institutions.

At the core of such a community would be concern for inclusive responsibility at both community and practitioner level. In 2002 *The Observer* (11 August, 'Scandal of NHS "Death factories"') reported the death of one elderly patient from dehydration. This had occurred over several days, with care staff not responding to his discomfort and not setting up a saline drip. Out of a sizable staff no one took responsibility for the patient. The assumption seemed to be that someone else was responsible, or would provide the necessary orders for treatment. An ethos that focuses on targets and orders is precisely one that can begin to erode the practice of responsibility – the target has been met, the order fulfilled, and 'Now I no longer need to care'. This is precisely why *phronesis* should be at the centre of reflective practice, to ensure that it is the fundamental *telos* that is being pursued.

Conclusion

In this chapter I have suggested that spirituality and ethics can come together in the caring community, a community that includes the professional caring communities but is always more than just that. By definition such a community is one that looks outward, to work with and share responsibility with others. It also is aware of the plurality within the community of care, seeking to value all the contributions and to develop and maintain effective partnerships. Such a community includes social, health and educational care.

As such, the community of care can embody the long-term commitment of moderated love. Yet it is always working its meaning out in the contract of the local situation. As such it offers to the client not just healing and health, but the associated values and ethos – in much the same way that the Olympics offers not simply the opportunities of sport but also the ethos of Olympism, embodying values such as fair play and peacebuilding (Parry 1998). The experience of the learning organization would suggest that such an ethos needs to be refreshed and renewed on a regular basis, in order for both the virtues of the community and the virtues of the members of the community to be developed and maintained. This is precisely the critical hermeneutic, focused by *phronesis*, that seeks to locate, critique and develop traditions of care, and focus the meaning in practice. Purpose, responsibility, and creative and collaborative responsiveness all come together in the professional ethos. Much of this is familiar to virtue ethics, but this moves beyond that in its stress on plurality, provisionality, and the stress on more affective and existential virtues, such as faith and hope.

The clients or patients then become part of that community (however briefly) and it is to them that I now shall turn in the next chapter.

6

Values, Virtues and the Patient

God grant me the serenity to accept the things I cannot change, the courage to change the things I can, and the wisdom to know the difference.

(Prayer from Alcoholics Anonymous (1976))

Introduction

In the previous chapter I suggested that the ethos of the caring community belonged to all who professed to care professionally. But how, then, does the patient fit in to that? Campbell and Swift (2002) suggest that to understand this we might think in terms of the virtues of the patient. In this chapter I will therefore be exploring values, virtues and the patient's part in the community of care. In the first part of this chapter I will suggest that moral and spiritual values are at the heart of the caring relationship, and that it is this relationship itself that is the basis for developing virtues in the client. Here virtues are not seen as goals of therapy but rather the fruits of the caring relationship – and, as such, critical to recovery. I will begin with an example from the world of counselling and psychotherapy, illustrating long term development of values and virtues in the caring relationship. I will then go on to suggest that the development of virtues is directly related to the development of autonomy. Finally, I note that it is possible to practise and develop virtues through particular techniques, which are best set in the spiritual and moral reflection of the caring community.

Moral values in counselling and psychotherapy

There are a variety of views on how psychotherapy or counselling should relate to beliefs and values. Richards, Rector and Tjeltveit (2003) note the increasing evidence that spiritual values and virtues can promote physical and psychological coping, healing and well-being, and argue that it is therefore important to make use of such resources in therapy. Rogers (1942), on the other hand, argued that there should be no attempt to influence the client, whose own particular values should be respected. Richards *et al.* (2003) accept that there should be no attempt to coerce a client but argue that the therapeutic relationship is not value free. Richards and Bergin (1997) note that because of ambiguity about the value agenda 'many therapists continue to implicitly advance their value agenda during treatment' (p.131). Hence, they argue for an 'explicit minimizing' style of the therapist, that is the therapist should be explicit about his or her beliefs and values from the start, and at appropriate times during their therapy. They argue that explicit communication of value is the best way to avoid covertly influencing the client. Some writers in pastoral theology suggest that this could even take the form of more directive counselling (Billings 1992), which assumes that the client is part of the same religious community and is thus simply being reminded of the moral meaning and discourse of that community.

Elsewhere (Robinson 2001), I have argued that in fact the moral basis of the counselling relationship is focused in that relationship and especially in the way that it embodies the core values of the community of care. The therapist embodies *agape*, empathy, *phronesis* and integrity. These deepen the classic Rogerian view of the counselling virtues or core conditions of counselling: unconditional positive regard, empathy and congruence. They provide an accepting environment within which the client can begin to make moral and spiritual sense of their experience, cognitively, affectively, and somatically. They also seek to enable the client to develop his or her own spirituality, working from the basis that spirituality and ethics can only be worked through in community – as exemplified in the following case study.

Case study

Diane had experienced a series of physically and emotionally abusive relationships as a child, each of which had tended to reinforce the effects of the other. Reluctantly Diane sought help from a counsellor, having found two courses of treatment with clinical psychologists unhelpful.

Initially, she found it hard to relate to the counsellor. She felt a failure having to come to a therapist in the first place and kept apologizing for being there. Diane assured the therapist that it would all be sorted out quickly, and would only need a few sessions. Along with this she exhibited real pain and exhaustion. It became clear later that she was experiencing severe flashbacks about the abuse.

In the first few sessions Diane also began to talk about her fears and concerns to do with work. She worked as a personal assistant to an administrator in a large health organization, and prided herself at sorting out problems. She looked after her boss, making sure he was not put under too much pressure. However, with changes in the organization there was increasingly great pressure on her boss and he was not able to cope. Diane took on responsibility for 'bailing him out', which often meant long hours at work and her own exhaustion. In turn, this made it less easy for her to cope with the volume of work. She was very bitter about the style of management: 'it is so unfair that I end up doing everything'. The stress was such that she was now losing her temper with colleagues at work.

Diane had no real friends. She no longer saw her father, and infrequently saw her siblings. She did try to keep in touch with her mother, but when with her never felt that she could do the right thing. When she was living in the family she had felt herself to be responsible for her brothers and sister, but had now given up on them. They never realized what she needed or what she was going through: 'I always had to do for them'. However, she still felt responsibility for her two nephews and niece. This was partly because she believed that their parents were not fulfilling their responsibility and that she therefore had to 'rescue' them: 'they never get a fair crack of the whip'.

For the first several sessions Diane alternated between realizing exactly what she needed, and deep depression. Usually she would articulate the first of these just before the end of the session. 'I know it sounds crazy for a woman of my age, but all I think I need is a hug… You must think I'm so strange'.

Diane began to reveal the spiritual and moral meaning that was at the centre of her world through the articulation of her narrative. Initially, this was narrative designed to disclose a view of her self that was acceptable or good. The therapist did not need to feel pity for her, or see her as weak or dependent. She felt pain but it would soon be 'sorted out'. Part of this initial presentation was a concern also to encourage the therapist to collude in a kind of magical spirituality. She consciously said that she was placing faith in her to sort this out quickly. Literally she was hoping for a parent figure – who would take responsibility for getting rid of the pain.

At the core of Diane's spiritual and moral world was a concern to defend the self and the values that gave her identity. These were based around a conditional ethic that stressed the need to please, to be self-sufficient and, to maintain the highest moral standard (moral perfectionism). This led to affect shame (shame at expressing feelings, especially anger) and need shame (shame at accepting of expressing needs). Alongside these was a strong sense of altruism and responsibility for others, such that Diane took responsibility for those she saw as vulnerable. As a result she had few boundaries and little skill in negotiating responsibilities.

Narrative articulation: Finding a voice

The articulation of her narrative enabled Diane to gain the necessary distance to begin to listen to herself and see the life-meaning she had developed. First this enabled her to begin to see the truth that had been obscured by that meaning. She began to speak of the painful incidents in her childhood and even discovered that one image that she thought was part of a compulsion to self-harm was actually a memory that she had repressed.

Second, the more that Diane rehearsed the reality of the past the more she began to see herself as an ambiguous figure. Prior to this she was a person who had failed. What went wrong was not the fault of her parents. Far from it, their action simply confirmed that she was unworthy. Now she began to see herself as someone who was responsible for her parents but also a victim. This was further underlined by the intensity of the pain she experienced.

Third, as she shared this, Diane began testing out the faithfulness of her carer. The therapist still remained there for her, despite the revelations: 'which you must find disgusting'. The level of shame felt was such that she asked her therapist to avoid eye contact. At this point Diane also raised, tentatively but seriously, her perceived need to be hugged. She knew the problems this might create in any therapeutic relationship. She and the therapist negotiated a contract that involved the therapist holding Diane's hand when she felt that she needed support.

Clarifying meaning

At one level Diane thought herself different and strange, a view based upon the shaming attitudes of her parents. At another level she did not have a real view of the world or her self precisely because she was too close to her parents. She had no identity separate from their 'presence' and from a life script that demanded her service and her silence.

Diane could only begin to find the distance and work out her separate identity through continued articulation, and in particular through facing up to and handling the ambiguity and conflicts that emerged from the narrative. A key to this was the development of a dialogic self so that Diane could hear and see herself as 'other' and begin to engage her self in dialogue. The role of the therapist was critical in enabling her to see the contradictions emerging in the narratives and then in giving her the space and the confidence to work through those contradictions herself. As she saw herself in the past the moral judgment was replaced gradually by a different perspective on her self. This was a very different self that she saw, one that called for a different moral response. Difference, in itself, had been seen as negative by Diane. Now it became something that she could engage with and make sense of.

At one level there was a development of shared moral meaning between Diane and her therapist through their initial contract, which set out expectations of the relationship, frequency of meeting and so on. At another level an affective moral contract was being worked out through the relationship itself. A striking example of this was Diane's affect shame, which meant that it was very hard for her to express anger, either about her parents or towards the therapist. She expressed hidden anger through sarcasm, which seemed once more to be testing the response of the therapist. A critical moment occurred when the therapist was late and for the first time Diane expressed explicit anger. She was able to express this because the therapist had transgressed the original contract, which set down punctuality as an important part of respect, and made this very clear. Diane's initial challenge was quite clumsy because she was fearful that it would lead to an adversarial response from the therapist. However, the careful, non-judgmental response from the therapist reinforced the nature of their relationship, validated the feelings and enabled Diane to reflect on and develop the skills of challenge. She was experiencing the possibility of criticizing another and still being accepted, the core dynamic of the critical hermeneutic. Eventually, Diane's shame could be returned to its origins as she rehearsed anger at her parents.

The more she expressed the affective level of moral meaning the more Diane could then begin to discern other elements of meaning that had reinforced her moral world. In particular, she had a strong Christian faith, which she felt condemned anger and offered a strong view of the family, not least with the command to honour parents. Once again this involved Diane in development of criteria with which to critique the church's use of such ethical principles, and confirm the real meaning of them. Hence, through cognitive work Diane was able to recognize that honouring did not mean unquestioning obedience.

New meaning

As the therapy progressed Diane began naturally to reflect on the spiritual and moral meaning of her life. This was partly because she had to replace the old spiritual and moral mantras that she had lived by, and partially because this is a function of human need. In noting this spiritual reflection as a part of psychotherapy Kaufman (1980) writes of, 'the need for meaning in life, for a sense of purpose to what we do, that quest for belonging to something greater than oneself, the search for significance which springs from the identification need' (p.136).

For Diane this led to four key areas of change:

- First, she had to work through to a new and explicit moral and spiritual meaning that had self-care at the centre. The old view had care of others as always being more important than care of the self. This was a process of learning, with strong affirmation of Diane's self-worth from the therapist and with attainable self-care objectives developed, the outcome of which would be reviewed.

- Second, Diane began to work on specific principles to replace her old ones, focusing on the meaning of care and love.

- Third, and closely connected, was the development of new purpose through rehearsing the negotiation of responsibility. As the responsibility was negotiated so she was able to see an effective and significant role for herself that did not depend totally upon herself. With this she began to lose her aggressive pride that believed that she could achieve all that was being demanded of her, and develop a firm humility – recognition of reality and of her strength and limitations.

- Fourth, as a result of all this, Diane began to question her beliefs about God. He had been seen as a judging and demanding God who had to be appeased, which reinforced her perfectionist and affective shame. She now began to view Him more as accepting and concerned for her. More importantly, she began to develop a real sense of his presence and with that a spiritual discipline that enabled her to find space for herself on a regular basis. In turn, this enabled her to attend church and to feel that she belonged there. Prior to this, her view of God and the church had been largely cognitive. There had been no sense of existential engagement. In effect, Diane was learning the meaning of faith for the first time. Prior to this religious faith meant giving assent to a good idea. Now it was about accepting dependence upon an other.

Other people return to, or rediscover, a faith in different ways. One abuse survivor quoted by Hilary Cashman (1992) writes:

When I was little no one mothered or cuddled me, but I used to stay with relatives on a farm, and I would go walking among the round green border hills. I felt as if these breast shaped hills were mothering me, and the earth warmed me. When I was little I would lie on the ground and cuddle into the earth and listen to the trees. I got mothering from the landscape then, and I do now, and that's where I feel closest to God. There I have no doubts about my faith. I feel held, but not healed. Something is holding onto me while I am going through the pain, but it doesn't lessen it or shorten it. (p.86)

It is important to note that Diane's move forward into new meaning also meant letting go of the meaning of the old world – of her polarized view of others, of the magical view of her parents and the fervent hope that they might change and suddenly provide for her needs. This partly involved Diane in a process of bereavement.

Response

Diane's new values and meaning now had to be embodied in action. In one sense without a confrontation with the past effective closure could not happen. This brought Diane face to face with crucial questions about how to resolve the relationship with her parents.

Initially, Diane had been unable to think about any sense of resolution not least because her view of Christian morality got in the way. She viewed the Christian gospel as commanding forgiveness for the enemy. The dynamic of command simply set up a new standard for her to achieve and when she could not do so she felt further shame at failing to achieve what the church wanted. In accepting this command as the word of the church, Diane, of course, was not taking responsibility for principles or the spiritual world behind them. She put all responsibility onto the church. Hence, for Diane at the outset of the therapeutic process there was actually no understanding of what forgiveness might be in context, or whether there were exceptions to this command, or how forgiveness might link in with justice and so on.

Thus working through to a creative response only became possible for Diane once she had worked through meaning at a feeling and conceptual level. With a developing faith in her self and in others she was able to let go of her parents. She saw that she shared a common humanity with them, and with that went away the power that had kept her in a silent prison for so long. They were no longer people upon whom her very self depended. She could let go and still live. The recognition of common humanity also enabled her not to seek 'revenge' or want to destroy her parents (Smedes 1998).

Nonetheless, the awareness of the truth demanded that her parents be held accountable for what they did. Once again then Diane had to work through very different, often perceived as contradictory, demands: a hope of offering forgiveness (taking the initiative in building a bridge) and also a concern for justice. Reflection on her Christian faith confirmed that both were important. She felt she had to both be open and also to challenge her parents. Forgiveness meant acceptance of what had happened and justice meant asking the abuser to account to her for why this happened. 'I just want to know why he did this thing. I want him to tell me.' In the event she finally was able to confront her father, whose response was one of contrition, which Diane accepted. However, this did not lead to reconciliation. Rather, it effected a closure and she did not see her father again. For her, that was resolution. She chose not to seek justice through the law.

In therapy like Diane's alongside issues of justice and forgiveness comes an embodiment of spirituality in the formation of new lifestyles. This is focused on new spiritual disciplines that enable self nurture and new relational networks that enable collaborative activities and so on. It is precisely through this final phase that the patient begins to fully experience hope, both in the sense of developing a ground of hope beyond the self and in the sense of having the capacity to envision the future and to plan for it in a realistic and creative way.

The therapeutic process

Finding new spiritual and moral meaning were at the heart of the therapeutic process for Diane. She brought her own beliefs and values to the process, began to gain distance through telling her story, and began to assess and critique her current meaning structures. She did not magically change, and spent a long time testing out the moral environment. Eventually, she did begin to articulate and practise new life-meaning and went on subsequently to look at finding ways of maintaining that, through the development of friendships.

The challenge to Diane's old life-meaning came through dialogue that had cognitive, affective and somatic dimensions. Above all, however, this was a challenge that Diane herself was enabled to make. The therapist, doubtless, could have confronted unhealthy client values (Richards *et al.* 2003). However, the most effective challenge came through Diane being given the space to deal with the dissonances that emerged, both within her story and within the therapeutic relationship itself (Halmos 1966). The client learns to take responsibility for what is in effect a process of developing a critical hermeneutic in her life. Such a hermeneutic is not just about ideas but about the client's relationships with the significant persons and groups in his or her life.

For Diane the process was also lengthy because she tried to find ways of avoiding responsibility for her own thoughts and feelings, something very understandable given the level of risk it involved to move beyond where she was and to reach out to herself and her parents.

The virtues

If Diane had been developing new values, through articulation and practice, she was also developing virtues. As discussed earlier, it is possible to see virtue as being exemplified within stories (McIntyre 1981) or modelled by members of a community (Cooper 2002). In both cases, virtues seem to be the goal of the exercise. 'Here is the example of the virtue, now you must follow it.' However, the case above suggests that virtues are not qualities that are to be transmitted through story, or given by one person to another, but are rather gifts of the loving dialogic relationship itself. They emerge from, and empower, the process that enables the person to see things differently, relate differently, and build up a very different moral world. The virtues are learned through a complex and rich dialogue that enables reflection, testing, challenge, and practice. The method is, in essence, person centred, taking seriously the virtues and values of the person, the truth of her spiritual environment, and enabling her to take critical and practical responsibility for both. This involves elements of modelling, testing, practice and habituation. Central to all this is development of a reflective discipline.

Each of the major virtues develop naturally from the therapeutic relationship, as described below:

Phronesis

The articulation of, and reflection on, the client's story enables the distance necessary for the client to see their purpose and values. The process, *pace* Aristotle, is of course more than an intellectual one. In order to gain that distance and reflect on *telos* the client has to work with the feelings that have kept the previous values and purpose in place. Moreover, *phronesis* is not a simple reflection on settled purpose, but involves (as Diane's care shows) a development and deepening of purpose over time.

Empathy

Diane could not begin to truly see herself or her family, largely because of the shame she felt. Hence, she thought of herself as being strange, both different and morally unacceptable. Once she began to see herself as both responsible and victim then she had to deal with conflicting feelings of disgust and care. The more she wrestled with and began to understand these, the more she could move into an empathic perception of herself, which could eventually see herself as not being responsible for the abuse. This was dependent upon a caring environment in which she felt able eventually to share and accept need. She, too, began to gain empathic distance from her parents, such that she saw that they were neither monsters nor perfect, but real, ambiguous people. The therapeutic relationships itself also embodied this with Diane coming to see the therapist as not a magician but someone with care, expertise and limitations.

Integrity

In one sense Diane already had strong integrity. Her values were strongly held and she was not afraid of letting people know about them. However, this had led her to be very judgemental of her colleagues who did not reach the standards she craved to fulfil. However, her integrity contained no sense of the integration of values and feelings, no capacity for learning, and no determination to take responsibility for her thoughts and feelings. The therapeutic relationship enabled all that to begin, and so set in place a development in Diane's values.

Patience

From an initial desire for swift solutions Diane built up the patience to stay with the relationship.

Courage

In some respects courage was being learned throughout the whole relationship. It took courage for Diane to begin to articulate her story. Eventually that courage showed in her capacity to challenge the therapist. Finally, there is the courage she showed in developing new values and new practices, and in seeking resolution.

Temperance

The third Aristotelian virtue was developed by Diane as she gradually learned not to react unthinkingly to crises such as her boss's problems.

Humility

For Diane the admission of her limitations was an admission of failure. Developing humility was critical in enabling her to accept need and begin to work within her limitations. This then enabled her to begin to negotiate responsibility.

Honesty

Reflection on her feelings and thoughts increasingly allowed Diane to be honest. Developing the virtue of honesty, however, was not simply about being able to tell the truth, but about enabling Diane to work through the very emotional blocks that prevented her from seeing the truth about herself and others. Truth indeed through that process could, indeed, then begin to set her free.

Diane had become, through the therapeutic relationship, part of the community of care. Through that relationship, and not simply through the practice of virtues, she was able cognitively and affectively to understand the moral meaning of the community and begin to practise that meaning. The result was the development of virtues that were essential to her recovery. At the heart of this was the gradual development of *agape* and empathy. It is precisely with the growth of these virtues that in some contexts the patient is then able to offer support or care to the carer, through the development of mutuality (Campbell 1984; Griffin 1983).

As Diane's strength grew she also found an experiential affirmation of eros. Working through her response she began to find purpose and action that she wanted to fulfill for herself.

It is important to note that moral development in therapy is rarely smooth. The moral world of Diane was such that she constantly projected her feelings and values on to the therapist. At times this meant an assumption that the therapist was judging her negatively. At other times this involved her making judgements about the therapist and her competence. This led to an emotional and conceptual wrestling around moral meaning that was the opposite of the wrestling set out by Fashing and Dechant (2001). They posit wrestling against the tradition, and negative interpretations of the tradition. What Diane was wrestling with was care. Only by such wrestling could an appreciation of that care and love underlying it be approached. At one point Diane questioned the motives of the therapist, 'Why do you do this? It is just a job isn't it? You don't actually care about me do you?' This enabled a conversation about the nature of care in their context.

It is important also to note that Diane did not simply leave the old moral world behind. On the contrary, this would still resurface periodically. The big difference after therapy was that the development of phronesis and empathy gave Diane her a new ground from which to wrestle with the old values. In effect, phronesis, empathy and integrity developed through that process of wrestling.

I want now to give a little more space to two other virtues, faith and hope, which I will highlight for two reasons:

- First, they have often been cited as two of the three theological virtues – the other one being love. As Fowler (1996) and the positive psychology school (Miller 2003) both demonstrate, however, these cannot be confined to theology.

- Second, both faith and hope have a clear moral dimension, something often ignored in books on spirituality.

Faith

The development of trust is often highlighted as being essential to the therapeutic relationship. I would argue that the relationship itself can go deeper to examine grounds of faith, grounds on which values are based. Cantwell Smith (1998) defines faith as a

> quality of human living. At its best it has taken the form of serenity and courage and loyalty and service; quiet confidence and joy which enable one to feel at home in the universe, and to find meaning in the world and in ones own life. (p.12)

For Diane the grounds of her faith were in her family experience. She looked to find faith in her parents but instead was faced by conditional acceptance that promised but never gave her love. Hence, the real ground of her faith was in her self. She was the one who would get things done and who ultimately win back her parents' love. But, of course, the more she tried to please them the less they responded. She badly wanted parents who she could have total faith in – hence her frequent false hope that they would change. As a result she found it hard to place faith in others, especially if they had limitations. She also had a strong conditional Christian faith.

Faith, as we noted in Chapter 4, is a virtue that embodies unconditional love. The need to discover an other who one can have faith in is critical to well-being. Genuine faith is tested at several levels and is not simply a form of magical thinking or unthinking belief. Hence, the whole process of faith development culminates in the capacity to have faith in others and the self, and to share responsibility. Diane began to explore this through developing faith in her therapist. For some time she saw her as less than perfect, because she couldn't solve her problems speedily. However, the faithfulness of the therapist showed her that it was possible to have faith in an ordinary, limited other. This, in turn, helped her to stop looking for perfection in her parents, and to see them as they were. From this faithful relationship she was able to begin to put faith in others and develop a different, less demanding, faith in herself.

Hope

The virtue of hope is often not given much space in ethical reflection. However, it is a key virtue in the empowerment for change, and thus repays a more detailed analysis.

For many people the idea of hope is about the giving hope to someone and about the ground of that hope. The narrative of hope here is brought *to* the situation. Two examples of this are theological hope and medical hope. The first of these is often expressed in terms of the resurrection of Christ. This provides the ground for hope, for salvation now and in the future. Hence, salvation figures highly in the care of the dying by the Christian church. The medical hope is often expressed in terms of the medical model. Here the hope is placed in the action of an other, the competent doctor or therapist. In each case there is a clear outcome – salvation and health – and faith in the outcome gives us hope. Hope in this sense is future orientated.

Hope, however, is more complex than a passive acceptance of the work of the other, and involves existential as well as doctrinal dimensions. Hope is about the capacity to envision and take responsibility for a significant and meaningful future. As such it is distinct from a generalized attitude of optimism. The experience of hope develops in and through the counselling or broader caring relationship, and the language of hope emerges from the dialogue and reflection on that experience. The development of hope links to other virtues, as we will now investigate.

GROUND OF HOPE

The primal ground of human hope lies not in the future but in the present and above all in an other. Many people have a sense of being hopeless in themselves. They feel this largely because they have internalized the explicit or implicit judgement of significant others. The ascription 'hopeless' actually means that they have no value, and therefore by definition have no future.

Indeed, for many the future simply involves the repetition of patterns of behaviour that always fail to achieve their goal of being accepted (Robinson 1998).

The need here then is for the person to feel a significant sense of hope in the self, something that can only be supplied by the unconditional acceptance of an other. This is forcefully put across by Henri Nouwen (1994) who notes the possibility of hope in a patient even when close to death, a hope dependent upon the presence of an other and needing no time to generate:

> But when a man says to his fellow man, ' I will not let you go. I am going to be here tomorrow waiting for you and I expect you not to disappoint me,' then tomorrow is no longer an endless dark tunnel. It becomes flesh and blood in the brother who is waiting an for whom he wants to give life one more chance....
>
> Let us not diminish the power of waiting by saying that a life-saving relationship cannot develop in an hour. One eye movement or one handshake can replace years of friendship when man is in agony. Love not only lasts for ever, it needs only a second to come about. (p.67)

REALISTIC HOPE

Hope, as Lester (1995) notes, cannot thrive on deceit or untruth. For Diane, hope was attached to the attempts to please her parents. But it was not a hope based in the parents, but rather a conditional hope based in herself being able to win them back. The whole basis of this was a distortion of the truth and thus a false hope. The generation of hope thus demands that the truth be arrived at through empathy, with all its ambiguities and limitations. The development of empathy and *phronesis* thus becomes critical for hope, not least with phronesis's openness to past, present and future.

Through such openness false hope can be identified and released. The acceptance of limitations also involves the development of humility. Humility has often been connected to a low sense of self-worth, quickly taking on a negative view of the self. In fact, humility, as noted earlier, is properly characterized as the capacity to 'have an accurate opinion of oneself. It is the ability to keep one's talents and accomplishments in perspective... to have a sense of self-acceptance, an understanding of one's imperfections, and to be free from arrogance and low self-esteem' (Tangney 2000, p.72).

Diane's perfectionism was a real block to any sense of hope, because she could never reach her own high standards and thus never be satisfied. At the same time she held on to a false sense of pride: 'Just give me enough time and I will sort it all out. I have to sort out everybody else's problems'.

Snyder (2000) suggests that the development of hope as a real virtue depends upon three factors:

- goals
- pathways
- agency.

GOALS

The capacity to hope is generated through a sense of morally significant purpose. Such good hope provides meaning which affirms the worth of the person. Hence, hope in those who are dying can be embodied in their concern for right relationships with significant others. In the light of such purposes realistic goals need to be set out. Hopefulness develops on goals that can be achieved. Hope may be a major virtue but it needs specific aims for it to be meaningful, aims worked through in dialogue.

PATHWAYS

Hopeful thinking looks to find ways to achieve goals. This involves a development of the creative imagination to be able to see what ways forward there are. This is enabled through the development of method and through practice, not least the widening of possibilities through negotiation of responsibilities.

It also demands the development of wisdom and empathy. Empathy is important in enabling the person to be aware of the possibilities in others. Wisdom means remaining open to the future. The use of imagination enables a person to project future narratives and work through different possibilities – something further facilitated by a clear method of decision-making. Snyder (2000) notes that hope is associated with the development of multiple pathways. Such pathways increase through collaborative work with others, which is enabled as resolution and shared responsibility is achieved. Through this real possibilities began to emerge and a feeling that things can be done further fuels hope.

AGENCY

Hope centres in the experience of the person as subject, capable of determining and achieving the goals he or she looks to. This is achieved to begin with through the development of the narrative and its related skills. In particular, hope is generated when a person finds she is able to own and take responsibility for the feelings, of shame and fear, that have dominated her life.

It is also achieved by the owning of values, the development of one's own method of decision making and by the practice that demonstrates the capacity to respond creatively to another.

Hope, thus, has several elements. It is not a discrete virtue but one that is gradually developed along with others. It depends upon several factors including method, reflectivity, process and dialogue. At its base, hope depends upon the discovery of faith in the other.

The inspiring of hope has been described by Pipher (1996) as the practitioner's first duty to the client and a major contribution to treatment. The contribution is summed up by Yahne and Miller (2003) as 'combating hopelessness by strengthening the therapeutic relationships, inspiring expectations of help and recovery, awakening emotional responsiveness, providing new learning experiences, enhancing a sense of self mastery or self efficacy, and affording opportunities for rehearsal and practice' (p.224).

Several points should be emphasized in from this review of hope:

- First, the development of virtues is ongoing. Virtues are never 'complete', and, indeed, can diminish. The comparison with muscles is apt. These can be developed but unless they are used regularly their power is not maintained.

- Second, learning the virtues involves cognitive, affective and somatic learning. The virtues can be explicitly discussed, as action is planned or values developed. At the same time the emotional content of virtues is engaged.

- Third, the somatic element is critical. The simple, consistent physical presence of the therapist can communicate attention, commitment, appreciation, and empathy. Many clients pay close attention to those physical cues of meaning and value. This reinforces the point that meaning is created in the physical context of relationship, including the wider environment of care.

  This all enables the development of a virtue vocabulary. Such vocabulary can be developed through reflection on the moral vision. As Meilander (1984) rightly reminds us virtues do not begin to make moral sense without a moral vision which they serve. This vocabulary can also be developed through reflection on the therapeutic relationship. Good examples of this were Diane's questions on the nature of the caring relationship, and subsequent reflections on her challenge of the therapist, how this felt and what it meant, e.g. in terms of courage. At the same time this, and the development of a contract, involve the practice of *phronesis*.

- Finally, learning the virtues needs the support of others – be that in terms of modelling or, more importantly, in terms of providing the community of care in which they can be developed. The client, in effect, becomes part of that community of care.

Autonomy

Much of the argument against therapists getting involved in belief and values of the client are based on the premise that this will endanger the autonomy of the client. The conclusions of this chapter are, instead, that autonomy can only be developed *through* attention to beliefs and values. Autonomy, seen as 'mastery of the self, the ability to decide for oneself' (Wilson 1999, p.7), has to be defended from coercion or manipulation (so called 'negative freedom'), but as a capacity it also needs to be nurtured. This demands precisely the environment that allows the person to be aware of their underlying purpose and values, developing what O'Neill (2002) refers to as principled autonomy, or moral freedom. It is precisely the development of the virtues that enable such an autonomy to be practised. Hence, as Tawney (1972) stresses, 'the seat of power is in the soul' (p.46). In the light of a virtue such as integrity this suggests that autonomy is not a fixed state but a quality that needs to be continually nurtured and developed.

Spiritual techniques and the virtues

Virtues can also be developed intentionally, and increasingly spiritual techniques are being used to enhance therapy – and in some cases are central to the therapy itself. The tendency has been to see these as instrumental, i.e. means to a therapeutic end. Hence, there has been increasing research into the effect of what may broadly be termed spiritual practices on the therapeutic outcome (Marlatt and Kristeller 2003). However, these also contribute towards the development of virtues within a community of moral meaning. I would suggest that they are most effective when the virtues developed by these techniques are explicitly discussed. In that way the client will know the purpose and meaning that is applicable to therapy and beyond. To illustrate, I will look at three examples meditation, prayer and twelve-step programmes.

Meditation

Meditation is often associated in care work with relaxation. This is reasonable, given the physical and emotional effects, including:

- reduced oxygen consumption and carbohydrate and lactate production

- reduced adrenocorticotropic (ACTH) excretion, producing the opposite effect of stress

- reduced heart rate and blood pressure (Benson 1996).

However, increasingly meditation is also been recognized as being valuable in enabling the development of 'mindfulness'. Mindfulness can be summed up as 'seeing how things are, directly and immediately seeing for oneself that which is present and true. It is…a bringing of our whole heart and mind, our full attention to each moment' (Goldstein and Kornfield 1987, p.62).

Mindfulness involves the transcendence of thoughts and feelings, enabling both metacognitive awareness and interoception:

- Metacognitive awareness (Marlatt and Kristeller 2003) is the awareness of thought and how we think.

- Interoception involves physical awareness.

Mindfulness is in fact the virtue of holistic awareness. It enables both the development of the observing self (and thus awareness of the self and social and physical environment) and also an awareness and acceptance of impermanence, (the continually changing nature of life). Hence, the development of this virtue is not simply about therapeutic utility but can also relate to the ethical identity of the patient and thus to the virtues such as empathy. Marlatt and Kristeller (2003) suggest that this transcendence also enables the person 'to become more comfortable with compassion, acceptance and forgiveness' (p.68). It could be argued that it is precisely the development of empathy that broadens the awareness of responsibility for the self and the other.

Meditation has been used as a treatment in a wide range of conditions including heart problems, obsessive compulsive disorder and other severe psychiatric disturbances. Given the way in which it relates to thought and feeling it is perhaps not surprising that the focus on mindfulness is being used increasingly in Rational-Emotive Behaviour therapy (Segal, Williams and Teasdale 2002). Segal et al. (2002) note the importance of this technique in particular in enabling the development of new perspectives, and thus enabling the client to develop holistically, rather than simply reinforcing coping behaviours.

Prayer

Prayer and associated ritual has had similar effects to meditation. This is summed up in research on the effects of the rosary and yoga mantras (Bernardi *et al.* 2001). Both forms of prayer involve on average six breaths per minute, leading to 'striking, powerful and synchronous increases in cardiovascular rhythms' (p.1446). This kind of prayer can be 'thought stopping', a closing down of the critical reflective faculties and, as such, has often been associated with negative cult practices (Barker 1992). However, there are many kinds of prayer that can have a variety of beneficial effects. McCullough and Larson (2003) suggest five kinds of prayer that are associated with well-being: contemplative–meditative; ritual; petitionary; colloquial and intercessory.

Contemplative–meditative prayer focuses not simply on the development of mindfulness but also on the presence of the divine. As such its focus is a holistic awareness of the other. Such prayer is generally non-analytical, but can be used in connection with, e.g., the reading of holy scriptures to provide a new perspective of those texts.

Ritual prayer can simply involve repetition of well-known words. However, ritual prayer tends to be part of public worship and this also builds up awareness, in this case of the community. In a ritual such as the Christian Act of Holy Communion it also develops further awareness of the presence of the divine lived in practice – in this case in the practice of Jesus before his death. The Communion service in one sense reenacts the story of the last supper thus enabling community members to identify with Jesus, and also reinforces the moral and spiritual meaning central to that community, in this case focusing very much on *agape* and empathy.

Petitionary prayer involves prayer about specific needs. This is often associated with times of crises and pleas to the divine to solve what seem to be intractable problems. This might be seen as involving a child-like response rather than developed spirituality. However, the reality of crisis is that it does take the person back to early feelings of fear and vulnerability. It is thus natural that these fears should be shared as part of prayer life. Sharing such fears can also help the development of mindfulness and enable the development of humility in the sense of accepting one's limitations and needs.

Colloquial prayer involves informal conversation with God. It can include conversation about anything, and is associated with increased intimacy with the divine presence (McCullough and Larson 2003). Hence, this prayer involves an increased awareness of the divine other and an increase in empathy and mutuality. Such prayer can also involve an articulation of feelings and tensions as is the case in psalms in the Old Testament. Prayer can thus focus on relationship with the divine in the context of tragedy and dissonance.

Intercessory prayer involves a conscious focus on issues, practice, and other people, in the context of relating to the divine other, and often in the context of the ritual community. As such this promotes both the awareness of different stakeholders in the local and global community and of their needs. It does not simply develop mindfulness and empathy, but, also concerned with identifying responsibility, both individual and shared, and supporting those who may be responsible. It is therefore action oriented and relates strongly to practical wisdom, and the development of hope. It also enables reflection on responsibility for actions or relationships that can be helpful for the negotiation of responsibility later.

Clearly, all these approaches stress both a community of practice and regular discipline in prayer. Behind that is the assumption that unless such virtues are practised then the virtues will be diminished, once more like muscles. The key point with prayers is that they enable the virtues to be developed through relationship rather than in a mechanistic fashion. The relationship with God focuses on his caring nature – the ultimate expression of *agape*. As Spohn (2003) suggests, this both provides an existential awareness of love and makes the person praying aware of how this contrasts with his or her limited capacity for love. Both motivate the person to respond. The meaning of love still has to be worked out through reflection around purpose, meaning and response and prayers can also involves a wrestling with meaning.

Addiction, and the twelve-step programmes
If spirituality can be said to run through the therapeutic process then it is even more explicit in the long tradition of self-help groups who work against addiction. The so-called twelve-step programmes are central to self-help organizations dealing with issues ranging from alcohol addiction to overeating, the classic example being Alcoholics Anonymous. The twelve-step approach offers a clear spiritual perspective on both the nature of the problems and the way to recovery. Research demonstrates that these programmes lead to improved psychological functioning and to a genuine commitment to change, and that they work well in co-ordination with other forms of therapy and counselling (Tonigan, Toscover and Connors 2003). Focusing particularly on alcohol addiction, four elements in this involve a

spiritual dimension: exploring the causes of addiction; the spiritual beliefs in the programmes; spiritual practices; the subjective experience of treatment.

EXPLORING THE CAUSES OF ADDICTION

The causes of addiction are complex and interactive, and can include any or all of the following:

- *Physiological and psychosocial factors.* Atypical metabolic patterns have been established in some advanced cases of alcoholism, though it is still not clear whether this predisposes the person to addiction or is caused by it. Compulsive personalities, or those who do not have effective ways of coping with stress, can also be predisposed to addiction.

- *Sociocultural factors.* Alcohol abuse, reflected in high abuse and addiction figures, seems more prevalent in certain cultures, such as Ireland and France.

- *Spiritual factors.* Clinebell (1990) suggests two key spiritual factors in the development of alcohol addiction:

  ○ First, for some the experience of alcohol is the equivalent of a religious experience. This involves using alcohol to 'feel good', to achieve a transcendence of the self.

  ○ Second, there is an idolatrous relationship with alcohol that looks to make it the foundation of faith. Alcohol consumption becomes the way of 'sorting out' problems, or trying to fulfil basic human needs, such a belonging or the need for security.

  In both cases there is development of a false spirituality which denies responsibility for the self and others and distorts reality, resulting in alienation from others. Behind both is a lack of purpose and spiritual meaning. Hence, Alcoholics Anonymous members speak of 'filling the empty bottle' – finding purpose and meaning that will replace the alcohol habit.

SPIRITUAL BELIEFS

The first spiritual belief expressed in the twelve-step programme is belief in a higher power. This is a very broad view of a transcendent reality, designed to be inclusive. Such an awareness is something that can be attained by most people. The Alcoholics Anonymous sees the God concept as being there in every person, accessed through reflection (Acoholics Anonymous 1976).

A second 'spiritual axiom' is the need to form a relationship with the higher power. At one level this about the development of a mechanism against relapse, with meditation and prayer providing a means of maintaining awareness of the other. Perhaps more importantly, it also sets out awareness of the limitations of the self and the need to rely on an other. Hence, there is a stress on the person herself as being powerless over alcohol (p.25).

A third axiom is the need for constant renewal. This accepts that there is no cure and points out that therefore the person must be aware of their needs and the danger of imagining that there is a cure (p.85).

A final axiom is the need to examine the self and to take seriously any sense of discord in the self. This focuses centrally on the integrity of the person and the need to remain constant to the purpose that they have chosen for their life. This leads to the practice of *phronesis*.

THE PRACTICE OF SPIRITUALITY

The spiritual axioms are reflected in the actual practice of the twelve-step programme. This includes:

- carrying out a fearless and searching moral inventory

- the articulation of the person's narrative, in the context of the AA meeting

- the embodiment of repentance, through seeking forgiveness and being willing to make amends. More widely there has been the development of forgiveness therapy (Sanderson and Linehan 2003). For some religious patients the practice of confession can be used for enabling forgiveness. However, for those with a high level of 'toxic shame' this is often not effective

- the development of mutuality in therapy with the person who has been helped becoming part of the healing community.

At the heart of such practice is acknowledgement that there is no point at which the person has overcome the problem of addiction and that she therefore has to commit herself to disciplines that will keep her spiritually focused.

The final two steps involve a deepening commitment to further self-examination and work in the service of others. Hence, this aims at enabling the development of a new purpose and value system.

THE SUBJECTIVE EXPERIENCE OF SPIRITUALITY

The subjective experience of the treatment process in addiction self-help groups focuses on three key virtues (Tonigan *et al.* 2003):

- *Humility.* Humility is learned throughout the programme, from the initial acceptance of limitations to the continual renewal of the self through making amends to others.

- *Serenity.* This virtue lies at the base of the AA prayer requesting the 'serenity to accept the things I cannot change'. The process enables the patient to accept the reality of her self and her situation. It also gives a sense of release at not having to face a purpose based upon conditional acceptance. Increasingly, serenity and the related idea of spiritual surrender, are being seen as important for other therapies (Cole and Pargament 2003; Connors, Toscova and Tonigan 2003).

- *Gratitude.* This develops both with the awareness of concern for and help of others, and also with release from debt and wrong doing.

Of course, the AA prayer also highlights wisdom and courage, and, arising from the relationships within the community, there is also *agape, phronesis,* empathy, responsibility, integrity, faith and faithfulness, as well as the Aristotelian virtues (see p.122). The stress on facing reality and resolving relational breaks caused by addictive behaviour also develops what Hauerwas (1984) refers to as 'peaceableness', the capacity to build peace.

Work with alcohol addiction then has spiritual and moral awareness at its centre. It does not have to be restricted to conventional religion, having a focus more on the person taking responsibility for herself and, through her awareness of the condition she is suffering from, taking responsibility for others. With that comes a critical change in spiritual and moral awareness, with the person learning concern for the self. Indeed, concern for the self is a key starting point for the programme, with a concern to change not for the sake of someone else but also for one's self.

This, then, leads to a renewal of identity and purpose and creation of a lifestyle that includes the development and maintenance of 'spiritual disciplines'. All of this is based on the person freely adopting the programme. Virtues here, once apart, develop from the relationships in the community of carers and from the explicit reflection on their meaning in practice.

Conclusion

In this chapter I have suggested that the client or patient is in effect invited in to the community of care, the same community that was outlined in the last chapter. How the client then responds to this is a matter for him or her. A brief visit into hospital, for example, may require little treatment, with no ethical or spiritual implications. For many, however, the ethos and values of the community of care will provide a framework of meaning that will be critical to their whole recovery, and longer term management of their illness. Once the client has begun to engage with values and taken responsibility for their life-meaning then he or she will move beyond the role of consumer to one of co-healer, engaging the whole self, and taking responsibility for their life. Titmuss (1970) had a strong sense of how health-care could enable the patient to contribute to the wider community of care through gift, and this could be part of a wider creative response. However, the immediate response available to all is to take responsibility for one's own health, and thus, where necessary, to begin to change beliefs, values and relationships. With the development of mutuality in the therapeutic relationship this can also extend to the patient caring for the professional. This can range from an expression of appreciation reinforcing the existential joy of the work, to an expression of concern if the carer seems stressed. In some cases, the client or patient can begin to offer a ground of faith or hope to the carer. This happens most strikingly in the care of the dying.

Virtues are involved in this therapeutic process. They are produced over time, or reinforced, by the healing relationship and, in turn, contribute to the therapy. The virtues are necessary in the areas that I have outlined above because a person's response to therapy and the development it involves can be seen as perceived risk, not least to that person's identity. The need for courage, empathy and so on becomes very real in that situation. And from that change come the responses to the ethical demands of other relationships, both new and old. In all of this the client lives out the critical hermeneutic, taking responsibility for the self and others, wrestling with the life-meaning he or she brings to the relationship, and sharing responsibility in creative development. Spirituality and ethics then become a vital part of the healing process which Swift *et al.* (2002) note includes even chronic illness such as arthritis.

In certain situations, however, it may be that belief has led to practice that is questionable. Does this still, then, involve enabling the critical hermeneutic or should challenge be more assertive and direct?

7

Challenging Faith

Genesis 22: a midrash[1]

And with heavy heart Abraham went to his wife Sarah and said, 'God has told me to take our son Isaac, whom we love, and sacrifice him as a burnt offering'.

And Sarah said, 'A shrewd move. This God is no fool. This is her way of testing you. What did you say to her?' And Abraham replied, 'I said nothing. I want God to know I will obey Him without question. I will do as He commands'.

And Sarah threw up her hands in despair and said, 'Abraham you are a bone-headed fool. What kind of a God do you think you are dealing with? What kind of a God would want you to kill your own son to prove how religious you are? Don't be so stupid! She's trying to teach you something: that you must challenge even the highest authority on questions of right and wrong. Argue with her, wrestle with her!' But Sarah's words smacked to Abraham of blasphemy, and he went into the mountains with his son Isaac.

And Sarah said to God, 'Sister, you are playing with fire. He is too stupid to understand what you are up to. He won't listen to me and he won't challenge you; if you don't stop him he will kill our precious son. Is that what you want?' And God said, 'Sarah, they have a long journey to the mountains; I'm hoping one of them will see sense'. And Sarah said, 'Like father, like son. You'll have to send an angel'.

And it came to pass as Sarah foretold, and the angel of the Lord spoke to Abraham the first time and told him not to kill his son. And Abraham sacrificed a ram as a burnt offering. And the angel of the Lord spoke to Abraham a second time and told him his offspring would be as numerous as stars in the heavens and would possess the gates of their enemies.

And the angel of the Lord spoke to Abraham a third time and said, 'Because you were ready to kill your own son in the name of your God you will be known as a great patriarch and millions will follow your example. And they will believe that He is indeed a jealous and a demanding God, and they will willingly sacrifice

---

1   Midrash is a Jewish term for a homily on a passage of scripture based on traditional Jewish exegetical methods. It usually involves an embellishment of the narrative.

their sons in His name and to His glory. And there will be bloodshed and slaughter in all the corners of the earth.'

And Abraham returned to his wife Sarah and said, 'God is well pleased with me for I am to be a mighty patriarch'. And Sarah said nothing. But she took the garments of Abraham and Isaac that were stained with the blood of the ram, and she carried them to the river to be washed. And the river ran red with the blood of generations to come, and Sarah wept bitterly.

And God came to Sarah at the water's edge and said, 'My sister Sarah, do not weep. You were right, it will take time. Meanwhile hold firm to what you know of me and speak it boldly. I am as you know me to be. Many generations will pass and a new understanding will come to the children of Abraham, but before then I shall be misheard and misrepresented except by a few. You must keep my truth alive'.

And Sarah dried her eyes and said, 'As if I didn't have enough to do.'

(Marion McNaughton[2])

In Marion McNaughton's midrash there lies a real power. First, it is centred around Sarah, Abraham's wife, and this changes the whole cognitive and affective landscape of the original story. We can now begin to feel something about a story that did not originally address the reactions of all the players. Second, there is a direct challenge of Sarah to God and to Abraham. God's method is questioned and She has in the end to take on board Sarah's suggestion of an angelic intervention. Sarah does not invite Abraham to think about doctrine but rather about the person of God. 'Is this really the kind of God you follow, who wants you to sacrifice your son?' But Abraham can't see beyond the challenge to his obedience. He is more concerned to please God than to think about what this will mean, to his son, his wife and himself. Third, the challenge comes from the base of a continued commitment from Sarah both to God and Abraham. That commitment remains in spite of the demands of God, Abraham's lack of awareness and Sarah's exhaustion.

Combined together, these features create a great example of moral imagination – the capacity to view the situation with empathy, and thus to see the underlying humanity. Sarah brings that humanity to the fore. Above all this midrash reminds us that nothing is beyond direct challenge, least of all faith.

Thus far it has been the contention of this book that ethics and spirituality have a complex relationship that is both about the way in which wider and

2   I am grateful to Marion McNaughton for allowing me to use this midrash. It is an unpublished piece of work that has had an immense influence world-wide.

holistic awareness informs ethics and about the development of ethical character and awareness. At the heart of this there is a wrestling with the critical hermeneutic, questioning our view of underlying beliefs and how they relate to any ethical decision. It is perhaps a short step from a critical hermeneutic to the more public challenging of belief. This chapter will begin to explore more fully how one might begin to challenge or enable challenge of belief in the context of the caring relationship. I will explore this through a series of case studies. However, I will begin by trying to place this issue in context.

The problem with belief

There are several reasons why most people are uneasy at the idea of challenging someone else's belief. To start with, few, including those in the caring professions, are specialists in this area and so most people can feel out of their depth when faced by a strong religious position that might conflict with good practice. Second, one of the basic moral foundations of care work is that there should be respect for the autonomy of the patient or client. This principle has even more weight in terms of someone's religious or spiritual beliefs. The right to hold one's own belief is also enshrined in law. The Employment Equality (Religion or Belief) Regulations 2003, for instance, makes it illegal to discriminate against an employee because of religion or belief. This also extends to students (Robinson 2004).

In many areas this regulation has been interpreted in very creative ways, looking to enable employees to practise their faith at work. The law also protects behaviour in some faiths that would seem to be discriminatory in the wider population. One example is the Roman Catholic Church's refusal to consider women for ordination. Such a practice is not subject to equal opportunities law. In effect the law has a conscience clause, allowing religious belief to trump equal opportunities. This practice of making faith safe from challenge has come to a head in the dispute over UK Roman Catholic adoption agencies refusing to place children with gay couples in early 2007. The Church argued that their genuinely important work should be allowed to continue, and their practice of not placing children with gay couples should be ignored because it arises from religious doctrines and beliefs. The doctrines in question were based on natural law which holds that homosexuality is a sin. In this case, however, the UK government has challenged the church's conscience and the equality law in the Equality Act 2006 takes precedence.

The respect accorded by law to belief is part of a broader philosophical and social movement to respect difference and particular faith positions. Nussbaum (1999) notes an extreme example of this with one anthropologist who argued in a conference that the introduction of the smallpox vaccination to India was wrong because it eradicated the cult of Sittala Devi, the goddess who up to that point had been responsible for healing smallpox. The underlying argument here was the need to respect diversity and culture, come what may.

In recent times the position of faith in public has become even more problematic with the debates about wearing the *niqab* (veil) or crucifix in public, and about the pictorial or dramatic representation of religious figures in art or satire, be that cartoons or opera. In the light of such debate it is not surprising that there should be a reluctance on the part of caring professions to challenge faith in an overt way. Part of the underlying dynamic that causes problems is precisely that the identity of a person may be founded in his or her faith. Challenging faith means challenging one or more of several things:

- the thinking process – its coherence and logic
- underlying value
- underlying doctrine
- underlying relationships
- underlying feelings.

Challenge in this context can easily be seen as a threat to the person and to his or her rights. Legislative and moral weight tends to encourage a view of freedom that is largely negative, protecting the person's right to hold whatever belief they want to hold. This does not help with any attempts to challenge belief. Such a challenge inevitably has to balance a number of things:

- the freedom/autonomy/needs of the individual
- the needs of and for the community – issues of belonging
- physical or psychological harm that might come to the individual.

One can see these principles emerging in the issue of circumcision. The Islam and Judaic faiths prescribe circumcision. In different circumstances removing with a knife part of the body of a baby without any medical reason would be seen an assault requiring legal intervention to protect the person and rights of the child. However, it is accepted in law that circumcision is a critical marker of belonging to these religious communities and thus the religious meaning and context of the act is respected. But where are the limits to such respect? Female circumcision is not legal in the UK and USA but is acceptable in other countries. It is also seen as a sign of belonging. It is a more severe procedure and inevitably is connected to the oppression of the girl. As Nussbaum (1999) notes, culture and religion can be used to legitimate reaction, oppression and sexism.

Inevitably then there are difficulties in framing a challenge to any religion or strongly held spiritual position. Nonetheless, challenge is important, given the potential for faith positions to cause oppression. It could be argued that challenge is part of any respectful approach to faith, precisely to see what that faith involves in practice. The first illustration I will use of how this might work in practice relates to Jehovah's Witnesses, where the basis of the challenge described is both to belief and to the consequences of that belief.

Jehovah's Witnesses

Jehhovah's Witnesses are a religious organization who see themselves as a restoration of first-century Christianity. They will not accept blood transfusions, based on their understanding of the prescription to 'keep abstaining from blood' (Acts 15:28–29) According to the conscience of the particular individual, they may accept derivatives of blood such as Rh Immune Globulin.

The major problem faced in medical care has been the refusal of Jehovah's Witnesses to allow blood transfusion either for themselves or on behalf of a patient who is a child. Faced by a refusal on behalf of a child, hospital staff will, depending on the severity of the condition and the need for blood transfusion, take the issue to the courts.

However, it is not possible as things stands to override the religious convictions of patients who makes a decision for themselves. Some Witnesses carry cards that set out a refusal of blood transfusion and absolve any doctor of any responsibility.

If a Witness willingly undergoes a blood transfusion then he or she would be excluded from the faith community, and could only return if there was repentance. In the year 2000 the Witnesses changed the rules on blood transfusions so that the Church would no longer take disciplinary action against a Witness who willingly and without regret underwent a blood transfusion. This has been wrongly interpreted by some to mean that Witnesses could now accept blood. However, the only change in fact was that no disciplinary action would be taken. In fact the Church would have no need to take action since the person concerned would no longer be accepted as one of the Witnesses because he or she was no longer abiding by a core tenet of the faith. Hence, the threat of exclusion still remains. Of course, if a Witness is transfused against their will, this is not regarded as a sin on the part of the individual. Children who are transfused against their parents' wishes are not rejected or stigmatized in any way.

Faced by such a refusal, how might a health professional respond? The basis of the patient's refusal is ethically clear. Witnesses do not intend to die, indeed they have a conscientious objection to suicide. They are, however, fully aware of the possible consequences of the refusal, including the possibility of death and are thus seen as competent to make a decision. Legal definitions of competence in this context are not affected by the nature of the belief, only by whether the patient is aware of the possible outcomes of the decision. Hence, one famous case saw a judge uphold a psychiatric patient's right to refuse treatment, even though the patient believed he was the world's best consultant surgeon (Kendrick and Robinson 2002). The patient was in Broadmoor hospital and was given a 15 per cent chance of survival without amputation of a gangrenous leg. Astonishingly he survived. For a Witness, however, there is the additional factor that their belief is the basis of a conscientious decision.

How then can conscience based in belief be challenged in such a way that the person is respected? Gillon (2000) argues that it is perfectly acceptable for doctors to challenge such a decision. The basis of this challenge is rational and can be seen, initially, as two-fold. First, the patient is invited to explore exactly what is meant by this decision. This would involve taking the patient through the decision-making process to check out if he or she understood the basis of this, and the consequences to themselves and all the stakeholders involved, including family, friends and work. If a Witness already has a card one might expect that they already have worked through this level of meaning. However, as Minow (2006) notes in another area of ethics, the simple question 'What do you mean?' is often not asked and as a result actions can be taken where meaning is assumed or obscured by different issues. Minow focuses on military ethics from Nuremburg to the Gulf Wars. She suggests that abuses committed by troops were rarely directly ordered. In most of the cases the order involved some oblique euphemism, that coupled with body language and the ethos of the unit, could easily be interpreted as negative. There may have been additional pressure from peers who viewed the victim as sub-human. Perhaps even more important was the ethos of obedience running through the Army as whole. In order to be, and remain, a part of the organization the trooper has to obey orders. However, as Minow argues, obedience does not preclude questions, and had the troopers actually asked their officers what they meant this would have provided an opportunity for clarification and transparency. Even such a question can be a major challenge to a negative culture.

The parallels for the Witness are close. Any Witness may feel pressured to follow a line because of the ethos of the community and because of the concern to continue to belong to that community. So decisions may be based around not so much the data of the situation as around the emotional needs of the person. In the light of that, the actual data may not have been fully digested by the person.

Gillon suggests that it can reasonably be seen as the doctor's role to work through this clarification. He notes that assuming a patient is likely to take offence is insufficient reason for not doing this. There are other situations, such as working through the nature and implications of mastectomies, colostomies or limb amputations, that might also offend. However, the doctor has to raise these issues, partly based on a concern for the best interest of the patient and partly to ensure that consent or refusal is fully informed. Asking patients to clarify and formulate reasons for decisions does not override patient autonomy – indeed, could be said to enable it. I would only add that chaplains and nurses in the discussion at some point could also usefully be included.

The second element in the challenge is that of ensuring the Witness is aware of the plurality of views within the movement. It is commonly assumed that an organization such as the JWs has simply one view on doctrine and its application. However, all religious groups have some form of plurality. In the case of the Witnesses, Gillon (2000) can point to a number of different papers that reflect different views within the group – in which case it is reasonable for the doctor or nurse to draw the attention of the patient to this plurality. This is not an attempt to coerce the patient but does give them more data at the level of doctrine and its application that might help them in making a decision.

The kind of debate within the Witness community is exemplified by Elder (2000) and supported by the non Witness Muramoto (1998). Both argue that blood transfusion has nothing to do with the 'eating' or 'ingesting' blood, which is what the relevant scriptures forbid. They claim this is further confirmed by the acceptance of the majority of Witnesses of medical injection and transfusion of blood fractions. Gillon adds that the vast majority of

Christians world-wide do not interpret the scriptures in this way. This makes it reasonable to ask why the Witness might hold such a different view.

Gillon (2000) also addresses the argument that to ask a Witness to consider opposing views and to justify their decision is against their legal or human rights. He writes,

> The claim is simply false. There are no human rights requiring the other to desist from asking one for explanations of ones beliefs or from requesting that one reads views contrary to ones own – assuming of course that 'request' *means* request and is not a covert term for coercion of some sort – i.e. provided that one is not obliged to meet such requests. (p.300)

Gillon adds finally, slightly tongue in cheek, that the reasonableness of initiating public discussion about beliefs and justification of beliefs is one that the Jehovah's Witnesses already fully accept in practice, not least through their frequent house visits and addressing of belief issues on the doorstep.

New Religious Movements

These approaches to challenge described so far are largely cognitive, and can be very effective, but point up an underlying dynamic for some religious movements that also have a strong affective domain. Simple challenging of doctrines on a cognitive basis can have the effect, as noted above, of challenging the very identity of the person, causing emotional problems. For the Witness this could lead to a defensive affective dynamic in which he or she responds to the perceived threat of questions by polarizing the issue, and thus avoiding any exploration.

In terms of Fowler's stages of faith (see pp.44–45) the approach of the Witness would be in stage three, where faith and related spiritual meaning is focused in the peer community. In addition, it could be said that the community does not generally inform the logical thinking of the person but tends to focus on the emotional identity of the person. This is seen at its most extreme in the 'cult' dynamic of New Religious Movements (NRM) (Barker 1992). NRMs are often seen as essentially negative. However, they do fulfil a number of needs, including those of:

- self-improvement
- self-knowledge
- self-understanding
- desire to make a difference in life/service

- sense of purpose and direction
- companionship and a sense of belonging
- structured community
- guidance
- sense of self-worth
- hope
- being loved and cared for/accepted
- feelings of power
- learning.

These are needs that any religion would hope to fulfil. However, the dynamic of the cult groups is to focus on the affective needs such that the member feels that these can only be fulfilled by that group. This is what lies behind 'love-bombing', in which the person is given great attention upon joining the group such that they feel unconditionally accepted. The strength of the bond is then tested by the group both in terms of ensuring orthodoxy of belief and through involvement in proselytizing. The continued love and care of the group becomes dependent on the person accepting the first and getting involved with the second. With that there emerges the reality of an exclusive and conditional community. Conditionality is, of course, associated with polarized thinking and thus we see the member of the 'cult' gradually turning his back on the other world and viewing the other as wrong, leading to conflict with families. Conditionality is related directly to the capacity to handle the plurality and ambiguity of the other. Hence, the cult member will tend to see the family as accepting the conditions or not, as either good or bad.

There is some evidence that new members join a NRM from another group based on conditional worth. For the late adolescent this is how the family is often seen, before epistemic distance can be achieved. In one sense, then, the cultic experience keeps the person in a form of late adolescence. The initial acceptance of the group, who does not even know the person, is seen as contrasting markedly with family life where worth depends upon academic or career success. However, far from a move forward this simply begins a new community of conditionality. Critically, the person has gained no epistemic distance from either group and are thus unable to see the limitations of the community, the plurality within their core community, or the ambiguity of any group. None of this is pathological as such: the person chooses to join, and their joining in fact may point to a strong sense of well-being. However, because of their affective dependence many may then find it very hard to leave. Hence, the autonomy of the person is radically curtailed.

The dynamics of dependence are also rooted in the perception of the leader of the NRM as the source of truth, and thus by extension the ground of faith. Hence, any exit counselling has to enable the person to gain epistemic distance from the leader, to see them as a real, and therefore limited and ambiguous, figure. It may be noted that different levels of this dynamic can also be seen in parts of all the established religions.

It is very clear in such a dynamic how the underlying faith of the person affects the perception of the other, leading to an inability to appreciate them. In turn this leads to a judgemental ethics, based around fulfilling conditions and rules. Challenging such a faith then may involve more than clarifying the intent and possible consequences, and encouragement to reflect on the plurality within the faith. It may need an encouragement to the patient to develop his or her narrative. This is not to focus on right and wrong but rather to help the person take responsibility for his or her perceptions. This may just be the narrative of childhood or family. The more narrative is enabled, the more value-conflicts will emerge. In the light of such conflicts it is possible to introduce reality testing. This involves helping the person to reflect on the basis of their perception of reality. For instance, does the perception of other persons in their narrative accord with the persons' actions and words? If there is a lack of congruence between perception and action then the attitudes and values that lead to that perception can be examined.

Another way to achieve this might be to explore with the patient any critical community to which they belong. A good example of this would be wider families and friends who are not part of the religious community. How do the siblings, grandparents, wives feel about this issue? In recent research (Backhouse, McKenna and Robinson 2007) on moral motivation and use of performance-enhancing drugs in sport it was noted that few drug users were influenced by moral principles. The strongest motivation to take drugs was peer pressure and the culture of the gym. The strongest challenge came from exposure to another relationship or network that had meant something to the person, setting up value conflict around a relationship. This is not unlike the dynamic in McNaughton's midrash, where Abraham is encouraged to look at the God who he has known and compare Her nature with what seem to be Her present demands.

Where there is time to develop this level of narrative, it would be possible to explore with the patient his or her responsibility over time. This takes the patient beyond the justification of decision now and invites him or her to consider the effect of withdrawing treatment, and thus termination of life, on a range of stakeholders over time. One effective suggestion is to invite the patient to think what he or she might say in a letter to his or her son or daughter once they reach their 21st birthday. This might involve feelings about this milestone, personal hopes and wishes, and possibly some explanation of why life-giving treatment was refused. Here, the professional carer could, in very affective terms, help the patient to engage his or her moral imagination.

These kinds of techniques have been used as part of palliative care, helping patients to focus on generativity – Erikson's term for contributing towards the next generation by performing meaningful work (see Browning 2006). However, they are also a way of focusing on the reality of the relationship in question, the affective importance of it and the responsibility of the patient to that person now and in the future. This can also be a way of enabling conversation with the patient's partner. Both may be part of the religious group, and because of that it may be that tensions which are there below the surface have not been allowed to be articulated.

In effect this looks to develop empathy as much as rational discourse, recognizing and responding to the affective dimension of relationships in the situation.

The mystique of conscience

Conscience is often given as the basis for respecting, i.e. not challenging, a religious ethical position. The Universal Declaration of Human Rights (article 18) recognizes 'the right to freedom of thought, conscience and religion'. However, it is not clear how easily rights language fits with the idea of conscience. The term 'conscience' has so many possible meanings that it is not clear what is the right that is being defended. Perhaps more importantly the term conscience can be used in this context in terms of negative freedom, the right to follow one's moral judgement. Aquinas (1981, Ia, q.79, a.13.) suggests that the conscience is the 'mind of man making moral judgements', and as such it cannot be given the kind of mystique that suggests that the judgement of conscience is either final or in some way independent of dialogue and debate. Historically, conscience has been seen as both rational (Aquinas's *synderesis*) and affective (St Paul's view of an interior norm free from legalism). My argument in this book is that ethics involves both and therefore that conscience should be seen in these terms. If conscience does involve affective as well as rational dimensions then it can and should be tested and contested, at both levels.

The mystique of offence

In all of this it is very hard to rely on the idea of offence as grounds for not challenging. As Haydon (2006) notes, offence is dependent on context. Moreover, any taking offence is an active not an automatic response. This means that the ground of offence cannot be assumed. The cause for offence could be anything from the fear that the challenge might affect the person's faith identity, to the fear that other members of the faith group might be offended. The cause could be well founded or irrational. Hence, there has to be some justification for taking offence, beyond simply the assertion of offence, in order to see if offence is reasonable. The argument that challenge causes religious offence comes close to the ancient fallacy known as *argumentum ad bacullum*. The *bacullum* is a stick or cudgel and the argument runs: believe me that this is an offence for me or else there will be a backlash. The backlash is, in effect, offered as proof of offence. It is precisely because of this potential threat that in 2006 performances of Mozart's 'Idomeneo', that involved representation of the severed heads of various religious leaders, were cancelled in the Deutsche Oper Berlin, though later revived ('Shelved Muhammad Opera to Return', BBC 2006). Of course, the problem with the argument is that the backlash does not actually prove that there are grounds for offence.

A respectful challenge that asks the person not simply what the faith foundation of their ethical position is, but also asks why he or she should take offence at such a challenge cannot of itself be characterized as offensive. Indeed, such respectful challenge actually helps the person to work through what the reason for the offence is. If a faith position is not able to survive reflection it is hard to see that it has much credibility. Sometimes, however, challenge has to be more assertive.

The case of Victoria Climbié

The second case study we consider moves us from an attempt to set up a critical hermeneutic, to a faith narrative that involved abuse and was not seen or challenged by a number of caring organizations.

Case study

Victoria Climbié was a child (aged 8) from the Ivory Coast who was sent by her parents in 1999 to live with family, first in France and then in the UK. The aim was to give her the best education possible. However, her carers in the UK subjected her to cruelty and abuse leading to her death. A key part of this abuse arose from an illness she had which caused incontinence. This was interpreted variously as wilfulness on Victoria's part and possession by an evil spirit. At one point she was kept in an empty bath tied up in a plastic bag containing her own excrement and forced to eat cold food. The Laming report (2003) noted that Victoria's relatives were members of the local church Mission pour Christ, and went to seek advice. The pastor advised that the condition was caused by possession and that it could be solved by prayer. Two weeks later the relative reported a brief improvement followed by a relapse. The pastor accused her of not being careful enough and thus allowing the evil spirit to return.

Several months later Victoria was taken to a second church. Victoria and her aunt disturbed the service and were taken to the crèche and given a drink. Though Victoria was shivering the church assistant did not realize that she was ill. At the end of the service the pastor spoke to Victoria's aunt and confirmed in his view the diagnosis of spirit possession, recommending that the aunt spend a week fasting.

Several days later the aunt reported to the pastor that Victoria had been unconscious for two days and had not eaten or drunk anything prior to this. At this point Victoria was admitted to hospital where she died. She was suffering from severe hypothermia, multi-system failure, and injuries too extensive to fully record.

The core problem in this case was that none of the agencies involved either effectively gathered the data about what was happening, or effectively challenged it. One doctor made a wrong diagnosis. Another concluded that there was abuse, but her subsequent communication was interpreted as allowing Victoria to go back home. The senior social worker was herself both black and religious, causing a reluctance to challenge those from a similar background. The church workers were dominated by the religious diagnosis and therapy. Hence, no-one was able to see behind the framework of spirituality built around Victoria by the churches, despite clear presentation of distress. It is likely that for Victoria it all began because of culture shock, leading to eventual physical illness. At no point was transcendence of the situation achieved that would enable the different stakeholders to look beyond the belief and value systems of the religious communities. The capacity of different agencies to challenge was also affected by the lack of coordination between the different caring agencies and the lack of any sense of shared responsibility. Ultimately, the responsibility for the 'case' was left with the church, and their care practice was not tested. Ironically, the only attempt to challenge was from the pastor's belief system in terms of how the initial religious prescription was followed.

A more appropriate social-care response to any such situations might involve two possible approaches. The first would be to engage the faith community in the kind of critical dialogue noted earlier. Following Canda's suggestions for social work (1989) this might involve:

1. Respect for the belief system. Without such respect it would be very difficult to enter a trusting dialogue.

2. Enabling a narrative, such that the full understanding of the practice and its possible consequences is worked through.

3. Clear communication of the ethical and legal values and expectations outside the religious community.

4. Clarification of any value conflicts.

Once again, none of this is about disrespectful challenge, and none of it is about asserting a particular moral view over another. On the contrary, it is about enabling critical moral consciousness in practice, thus enabling the different groups involved to look beyond their boundaries and be aware of the different belief and value structures. Had the churches been more aware of the health-care values in the UK they might have been less inclined to attempt in house, and unmonitored, responses.

Faced by such a case Beckett and Maynard (2005) remind us that the duty of those in social care is primarily to the child. In this respect a second possible approach here is not to see this as a religious issue, but primarily as an issue of care. This means making it a priority to determine exactly what the care and conditions of care involved. If there is suspicion of abuse, then issues of respect for diversity of faith take second place. There is a further parallel with cults and how they have been dealt with especially in universities (Robinson 2004). The most effective response has been not to question the belief or the culture, but the practice. Hence, where a student has been phoned twelve times in one day by a cult member this is taken as being harassment, regardless of any belief context. In Victoria's case it is her condition that should have been investigated. In addition any awareness of the practice of exorcism or fasting should have been investigated and challenged, purely because both involved psychological or physical risk. Hence, the core challenge here is reality testing, clarifying exactly what the practice and the condition means. Religion cannot be assumed to be benign.

Homosexuality, faith and mental health

In the first case study we highlighted belief and its effect on therapy. The second case study looked at abuse in the context of a belief structure and a context of fragmented responsibility. Our third case study focuses on mental health where the belief system can contribute towards the presenting problem but where there also may an issue of abuse – in this case homophobia – in the context of the belief system and broader spirituality.

The issue of homosexuality is a problem for many of the major religions including Islam. I have chosen a case from my experience in the Christian faith as an example of how such an issue can be at the centre of mental-health problems.

Case study

A student was admitted to hospital after an unsuccessful attempt to commit suicide. He was the president of a student religious association that had a very conservative theology. He was three months into the job and going through some pressure both in university work and in his family, when he began to have sexual feelings for another man in the student society. It took him some time to admit to these feelings, so shocked was he by them. His religious beliefs deemed homosexuality to be morally wrong, based on a reading of Christian scriptures, and the belief that God had created men and women for the purpose of procreation. He had also been to a school that had a strong aversion to homosexuality and was brought up in family that saw homosexuality as abhorrent.

In the context of such beliefs and feelings Paul found himself questioning his very identity, and as a result was deeply ashamed of his feelings. The subsequent crisis came to a head when after a drink he made sexual advances to the man he desired and was violently rebuffed. The man was another member of the student society and Paul was then afraid of being 'outed' and ridiculed. As a result he threw himself out of a third-floor window.

The nurse dealing with Paul listened carefully prior to the psychiatrist arriving to see him and sympathized with Paul's situation. She urged him to go with his feelings and to stand out against the homophobic behaviour. Paul had little understanding of what this meant, feeling only the shame of his homosexuality and the shame of having tried and failed to commit suicide.

Paul's shame was initially resolved by him through viewing the homosexual feelings as an illness – and therefore thus not a sin. He left hospital determined to find ways through his local church of being healed of this affliction. Accepting that his identity was threatened by something outside himself was Paul's way of dealing with the problem. This contrasts directly with the nurse's view that homosexuality was simply about sexual identity that was fixed, and that there should be no guilt attached.

The nurse had introduced Paul to the idea of plurality in the area of sexuality but had done it in such a way as to infer a strongly polarized debate. Far from enabling Paul to consider the various different positions on the issue and so begin to gain some emotional distance from it, Paul had felt forced to choose between the divergent views. To go with the view that homosexuality was acceptable and that his family and friends were homophobic felt to him like having to give up everything that had been important to him, and he simply did not feel able to do this. Because of this, his conversation with the nurse took place purely at an affective level, never examining the ideas or their implications. This meant that he was not actually looking at the reality of the situation, and above all not expressing and reflecting on his feelings. Hence, his judgement about values and beliefs were made without real awareness of what was happening to him. Clearly, helping Paul through this crisis would take time to work through the different aspects of his story.

Paul was part of a family that had a strong Christian perspective but in terms of family ethos gave the impression that acceptance was based on conditions. Several generations had been to both public school and Oxford University, and Paul had grown up seeing such achievements as competitions for acceptance by his parents and the wider family. Paul had been to public school but had then gone to a large university in the North of England, and he already saw this as letting down his parents. For him, achieving the presidency of the student Christian society was a key redeeming action. An admission of homosexuality via an embarrassing public *faux pas* would undo all this good work and be something of an ultimate failure, not least in a family where his two elder brothers were already married with children. Already then for Paul there were strong values, around conditionality, achievement, and identity that were being 'attacked' by what he had experienced. These values formed the basis of his spirituality, relating closely to his religious choice and to how he lived his life. However, the value 'battle' that followed Paul's experience in hospital was not articulated and thus not reflected on. Paul's underlying values formed the context within which he viewed his religion and the various doctrines. Hence, in terms of his Christian anthropology he had a very straightforward view that homosexuality was a sin against the creation purpose of God. The way to respond to the homosexual feeling was therefore to seek healing. This was reinforced by the strong conditionality that was his family experience. Hence, he left hospital with a conditional ethic reinforced and determined to get himself right with God – and ultimately with his family.

Ideally Paul should then have been given space to examine the context of his spirituality and the crisis of value that was at the heart of his attempted suicide. This reflection would have focused on the conflict and thus also on the actual feelings of homosexuality. This was a second area that Paul had not begun to explore. He had had girlfriends in his school and early student days largely to please his father, but for the most part these had involved surface attraction. None of this had meant that he was 'homosexual', anymore than his feelings of attraction to another man meant this. It did mean that in terms of emotional and physical relationships he had not begun to explore or understand the nature and strength of sexual attraction. Hence, the strong feelings for the other man were a shock both at a value and an affective level. Once again this all linked into his theology, with its emphasis on the need for physical and emotional control, and the dangers of inappropriate behaviour.

For Paul, exploring these areas required a safe space in his religion, but outside his particular church tradition. The psychiatrist had given him some time, and had then referred him to a counsellor. However, Paul saw a counsellor as a secular threat to his faith. In any case, an appointment with the counsellor wasn't available for two months. Instead, Paul went to see the university chaplain. Chaplains can be good examples of figures who religious patients can trust, but who do not reinforce narrow or conditional theology (Robinson 2004). In this case, the chaplain could help Paul work through the underlying value and affective issues and reflect on the different views that might exist within his religion and beyond, enabling him to transcend his belief and value system and assess it. In the same way that Gillon suggested that Jehovah's Witnesses patients might be referred to the examples of plural thinking within their tradition, it might have been possible for a doctor or nurse to do this in this context. It is important to stress that this is not a matter of trying to take the patient away from the community of faith, or turn his back on the good life, it is simply a matter of informing the patient that there are many different views within the religion, and asking if he is aware of these. For Paul it was more important to begin his affective situation as he experienced it and then to examine the different theological perspectives.

Theological perspectives

In Christian theology there are many different views on homosexuality and the debate still continues in different ways and in different contexts. Nelson (1978, pp.188ff) suggests four broadly different approaches to homosexuality within Christian theology:

- The first is the 'rejecting punitive' approach. This rejects the possibility of a theology that accepts homosexuality and has a punitive and condemnatory attitude towards homosexuals.

- The second is the 'rejecting non-punitive stance'. Famously set out by Augustine as hating the sin and loving the sinner, this argues that human beings only find fulfilment through heterosexual relations, and therefore homosexual practice should be rejected as against God's plan. It should therefore be condemned as practice, whilst at the same time remaining committed to the person.

- The third approach is 'qualified acceptance'. This sees homosexuality as against God's plans but accepts modern psychology's view that homosexuality cannot be changed. It is then a condition. The orientation should be sublimated and if that is not possible the relationship should be lived in an ethically responsible way, in fully committed relationships.

- The final approach is 'fully accepting', with an ethical focus on love and how this is embodied in different ways, rather than on the principles of natural-law ethics.

Trying to demonstrate a 'right' view amongst these four approaches is very difficult, not least because each use scripture, rational argument and tradition in different ways, and encompass a broad range of spiritual and cultural outlooks.

Merry (2005) notes a similar plurality in Islam, and calls for a re-examination of 'conceptual models and terminology' (Bilgrami 1992). Halstead (2005) recognizes plurality and thus the opportunity for real dialogue within the Islam. Nonetheless, he argues that the majority of Muslims globally would see the homosexuality as an 'abomination'. The same is probably true of the most members of the Christian religion. In America, there is real diversity of views about homosexuality, whilst the Christians in Africa are for most part negative. But even this denotes that as religions grow they are met by different cultures and thus develop many different voices. Once more this plurality is part of what it is to be an institutional religion.

In trying to work through these issues one Church of England document, *Issues in Human Sexuality* (1996), has tried to hold together the ambiguities at the centre of the issue. They affirm a natural law position, i.e. natural law argues that God created the world with a clear purpose and this forms the basis of morality. In this it is argued that God's purpose for humanity involves life-long heterosexual relationships. Such relationships embody long-term care – *agape*, sexual fulfilment, and the possibility of procreation. Of course, once this positive argument for heterosexuality is stated then there is the danger of seeing anyone who does not conform to this purpose as being wrong, and thus by extension as unacceptable. Even celibacy might be questioned.

There seems immediately here a difficulty about using purpose and aspiration as standard and thus prescription. The report gets round this by suggesting keeping natural law and the related practice as aspirational. The result is that it is possible also to affirm other kinds of behaviour, including life-long committed same-sex relationships. It affirms these whilst acknowledging that they are not part of God's purpose.

Three problems can be observed with the natural-law position:

- First, it assumes the model of single purpose and this is difficult to sustain, given that, for instance, there are three purposes enshrined in the Anglican marriage service – procreation, sexual fulfilment and companionship.

- Second, it is impossible to require that the procreative purpose be fulfilled, not least because some heterosexual couples cannot have children. Hence, it may be that companionship and sexual fulfilment are the only two purposes that can be achieved.

- Finally, there is the problem of the priesthood. The report argues that it is wrong for a practising homosexual to be a priest. The grounds for this are not clear. Some argue that this involves double standards, with no room to for qualified acceptance for a long-term single-sex relationship. Others suggest that this is really about recognizing the plurality of views within the church and the strength of those views. In the light of potential division it becomes critical to ensure that the leadership within the church is not seen as favouring one group over another. In a broader canvas this argument seeks to keep dialogue open with parts of the church – notably in Africa where homosexuality is vehemently opposed.

This is a good example of an ethical and spiritual dialogue that has no simple solution. It cannot be characterized as a simple matter of justice for homosexuals, because it involves different views bound up in doctrine, and very different cultures. In the light of that, commitment to others in the church requires a continual wrestling at all these levels. As one might expect in this context there are many arguments that do not really address the issues, or which are really fronts for underlying fears. The 'slippery slope' argument once more comes to the fore, to the effect that once accepted then homosexuality would erode the practice of heterosexual marriage, and thus change the moral base of society. As we saw with the conjoined twins argument this is fallacious. There is simply no evidence that this is bound to happen. It is also a mistaken view of social change, and indeed, of society. It assumes that a meta-narrative around sexuality could be sustained, whereas in fact society has a wide plurality of views. Change in society takes place not because we let go of a meta-narrative, but for many reasons, including social and economic. In light of this all that can be done is to wrestle with our different views and keep wrestling.

Homophobia

It can be objected that it is all very well looking at challenging dialogue and respecting plurality, but at the centre of much of the dialogue is simple homophobia and this needs to be challenged directly. Merry (2005) writing on the Islam perspective, suggests that there is militant bigotry in many of the Islamic values, and one might see a softer bigotry towards homosexuality in the particular Christian perspective on homosexuality that invites us to love the sinner but hate the sin. If sexual practice affirms sexual identity then it would seem impossible to split the two in this way, at least without an implicit condemnation of the person as well as the practice. In a very 'caring way', the argument goes, 'loving the sinner' reminds the homosexual that they are indeed a sinner, and thus this argument easily reinforces the negative views of homosexual orientation. Homophobia, soft or hard, should be challenged, so the argument goes.

However, even the use of the word homophobia in this debate needs careful handling:

- First, homophobia in the strict sense is an irrational fear of homosexuals. This is precisely something that needs care, not attack. Paul himself had a form of homophobia based around his conditional ethic, and it was important for him to explore these feelings and begin to understand why he had them. Hence, for him this was not about challenging homophobia in others, but challenging it in himself. The challenge could only be made by him through the development of empathy. This is the case for many people with homophobia. To simply condemn it, tends to lead to polarization.

- Second, there is the danger of using homophobia as an argument *ad hominem*. This refers to the fallacy that states that an argument is logically wrong because of the nature of the person. Hence, rather than looking carefully at the arguments that are set out against homosexuality and critiquing these as they stand, it is easier to dismiss the argument as the product of a homophobic person. Halstead (2005) wants to argue that it is possible to disapprove of homosexual practice without being homophobic. He suggests that homophobia be defined not simply in terms of fear but rather in terms of practice. Hence, he defines it as 'bullying, discrimination, abuse and social avoidance directed against homosexuals because of unjustified fear or hatred of them' (p.39). These homophobic behaviours are quite distinct from finding homosexual behaviour to be unethical. Conceptually this makes sense, but testing that out in practice needs careful attention.

- Third, it remains important to challenge homophobia where there is evidenced of this in terms of bullying, discriminating and abuse. In this context this means focusing on the action, not the feeling, and challenging that.

None of this is an attempt to assert the moral case for homosexuality, or to make a moral judgement about this. It simply acknowledges that the debate about homosexuality cannot be summed up simply in cognitive doctrinal terms. The issue is complex, involving a mixture of cultural, religious and psychological dimensions. Whilst homophobic behaviour can be challenged directly, the other agendas require careful dialogue that enables tensions to be worked through. Paul had to wrestle with all the different meaning that his religion, family and culture brought to this issue. This meant him taking all the arguments about different theological views and how they related to thought and feeling seriously, enabling the development of a critical hermeneutic.

One might think that such a challenge would lead to more confusion. But in fact it lead to greater awareness of the self and the place of different values and beliefs structures. For Paul this involved increasing acceptance of responsibility. He gradually began to take his own responsibility for his own thoughts and feelings, refusing to accept that they had to be determined by others. Then he began to work through his responsibility to himself and others. This included testing his responsibility as president of the student group. If he did determine that he was gay and chose to follow that path then he chose not to accept any responsibility for any effects this might have on that group. The same applied to his family. This led him to engage members of both groups in explorations about his sexuality. In doing that he received unexpected but not uniform support from both groups that further enabled honest reflections on sexuality.

At the heart of such reflection has to be an honesty about traditional views, that they could be wrong or inadequate. The only way of determining the validity of those views and thus respecting their authority is to test them honestly. In this respect Browning's (1983) approach to counselling is problematic. He wants the client to find the truth about themselves and meaning in life, and thus wants to respect autonomy, but is clear that there is a truth out there that he wants them to discover. Hence, he writes that 'pastors are inevitably leading their clients somewhere, even if only by silently drawing certain boundaries and eliminating certain options' (p.96). He notes this explicitly in terms of homosexuality, a phenomenon that he argues has no moral base either in natural law or consequentialist thinking. However, I would argue that it is not clear that these grounds provide sufficient justification to judge homosexual practice as morally wrong. More importantly in the dynamic of care it is precisely that thinking, and the related feelings, that should be tested. Open challenge will then enable a person to either accept the wisdom of the traditional position, or stand out against it whilst still respecting the community. This allows for much more subtle and responsible thought and behaviour.

In Paul's case he began to accept that he was homosexual. He realized that remaining in the presidency would be too difficult pastorally for many of the members and for the national organization. Hence, he chose to resign, but to remain a member of the student group and also to join a different church, where he was able to explore purpose, and work through resolution with his father. He still belonged to the Christian Church, but belonging no longer meant having to accept community doctrine in the same way.

Given the complexity of spirituality, both doctrinally and exisistentially, it is very hard to see how any doctrine can act solely as the basis for an ethical judgement. Doctrine can inform and even provides criteria for how moral responsibility is developed. Hence, for instance, an anthropology can help show the importance of mutuality and interdependence. But the doctrine cannot of itself determine what is right and wrong. This will always be contested by other different doctrines and affective narratives, and above all by the criterion of inclusive responsibility.

Conclusion

In this chapter I suggested that the public challenge of faith is necessary. The idea that faith of whatever kind can hide behind 'conscience' has little merit, not least because conscience should be open to the test of rational reflection. There is also little merit in trying to differentiate too starkly between religious and secular thinking. Any non-religious thinking includes spirituality of some kind and has to clarify this. Any religious thinking includes plurality and this will always question the idea that an ethical response can be built simply or solely on doctrine. Levinas, Bauman and other agapeic theologians all question this. The challenge of any faith position should focus on the practice, but should also take the faith seriously enough to test it against that practice. Where the practice is harmful it should be challenged on that basis. Where there is an issue of autonomy the client or patient should be enabled to focus on their own spirituality and responsibility.

This is not then a simple model of ethics wrestling with spirituality. It is about how values and beliefs are wrestled with cognitively, affectively, somatically and relationally. All of those values and beliefs are anchored in communities that give us faith and purpose. All of these have to be questioned, through the test of internal debate, opening out to the plurality within, and the test of plurality from outside these communities. The ultimate criterion of such challenges is once again inclusive responsibility. McNaughton reminds us that even, and perhaps especially, God is subject to this. There is a moral imperative to respectfully challenge faith in the context of care. Perhaps the most common challenge to faith in this context is focused in feelings of injustice, and it is to justice that the next chapter turns.

8

Spirituality and the Domain of Justice

The moral imagination requires the capacity to imagine ourselves in a web of relationships that includes our enemies; the ability to sustain a paradoxical curiosity that embraces complexity without reliance on dualistic polarity; the fundamental belief in and pursuit of the creative act; and the acceptance of the inherent risk required to break violence and to venture on unknown paths that build constructive change.

(Lederach 2005, p.29)

Introduction

In the passage above Lederach's (2005) argument begins to sum up the transformative ethics that this book has been outlining. He focuses on the sharp end of outcomes, and in particular on peacebuilding and conflict resolution. At the heart of that very solid ethics is the moral imagination. This is the act of empathy that brings the enemy into the community. Lederach (2005) does not suggest that that community is without blemish. On the contrary, empathy can enable us 'to be honest about the sources of violence in our own house' (p.34). This is part of what Browning and Ricoeur see as the being critical hermeneutic.

Then Lederach moves on to the creation of a new reality, reminding us that all realities are constructed. Hence, he urges us not to see the terrorist as a madman, but rather to ask how he constructs his reality, what is the spirituality of terrorism. From there the moral imagination moves into the creative response, enlarging what is possible. Spirituality, then, is there even at the heart of what we see as justice and injustice, the sharp and very public expression of ethics.

In this last chapter I will look at how questions of justice can pervade care, not in the sense of care policy (though this is, of course, connected) but in the sense of making meaning. I will then reflect on freedom and authority in care and how they relate to spirituality. I will end by issuing a challenge to religions to join in the narrative of care.

Justice and suffering

Justice as a moral concept pervades spirituality. It is there at the heart of suffering.

In that context, justice is often viewed in terms of meta-narratives, evoking questions such as 'Why has this happened to me?' By definition this event feels unjust, unfair, and to explain it I need to posit some framework of justice, against which we can judge it.

Religious approaches to justice have in the past felt it necessary to take that question very seriously. After all, an omnipotent creator who loves his creation might seem to operating out of character by allowing so much suffering. The most primitive approach was to connect suffering with justice as merit. Suffering was punishment for something done by the person or one of their forebears. If the reason for the suffering is not evident, then it was reasonable to assume that the wider picture, which we cannot see, but is seen by God, would contain the answer. Arguments such as these formed the basis of theodicies, attempts to reconcile God with the reality of evil and suffering.

This was expanded in later philosophy to the idea that suffering was part of an overall plan that was ultimately for the good of all. In this light, everything, even suffering, was for the best in the 'best of all possible worlds', a view elegantly undermined by Voltaire (1959).

Functional views of suffering can also be connected to a negative view of the world. Socrates, on the eve of his death, welcomes the end, because this will take him away from a world of change and suffering into a changeless world where all will be perceived clearly through the Forms or Ideals of Beauty, Truth and Goodness. Suffering then is ultimately not part of the real world, and can be borne, with the aim of moving beyond this world to the more real world. A similar dynamic can be seen in the spirituality of Hinduism and Buddhism, where suffering is seen as inevitably part of life. It can, however, be transcended in and through religious faith.

The Christian faith also took Jesus and his suffering as a way of finding meaning. He suffered and died in order to save, so the argument goes. But suffering is still instrumental, in which the salvation is conditional upon it. Hauerwas (1986) takes this further to argue that suffering, and the capacity to face suffering, is central to human experience and the development of empathy, and 'it is the capacity to feel grief and to identify with the misfortunes of others which is the basis of our ability to recognize our fellow humanity' (p.25). But even this runs the danger of making suffering instrumental and thus neither taking the sheer evil of suffering seriously, nor, frankly, letting God off. Hence, Weil (1977) for instance, suggests that some suffering, which she refers to as 'affliction', is irreducibly negative. There is no meaning or hope to be found in the experience of suffering which because of its intensity or duration reduces the person to an object. There is no Providence that will suddenly lift the suffering to meaning not least because, as Weil argues, God has set up a distance between himself and creation. Our task is to simply live through the duration of suffering along with more positive experiences that may, or may not, come our way.

Turning to the Old Testament, and especially the psalms, we find that suffering is faced head on. Meaning is worked through in the light of a faithful relationship. In the psalms the psalmist remains faithful to his god, but shares the pain and the blame with him. Breuggemann (1984) notes that such expressions of spirituality:

> lead us away from the comfortable religious claims of 'modernity' in which everything is managed or controlled. In our modern experience, but probably also in any affluent culture, it is believed that enough power and knowledge can tame the terror and eliminate the darkness. But our honest experience, both personal and public, attests to the resilience of the darkness, in spite of us. The remarkable thing about Israel is that it does not banish or deny the darkness from its religious enterprise. It embraces the darkness as the very stuff of new life. Indeed, Israel seems to know that the new life comes from nowhere else. (p.53)

If God is silent in some suffering for Weil how much more was he silent in the experience of the Holocaust. The agonizing question, 'where was God in Auschwitz?', still echoes. Levinas (1988) can see no theological narrative providing justification for suffering on that scale, suggesting that it is actually immoral to see the suffering of another as having a purpose. To look at another's suffering and see it as fulfilling a purpose is to see them as means to that purpose and therefore not to respect them, and their experiences, for what they are. This is another form of denying the reality of suffering, and the fact that it can have no obvious meaning. He also adds that there can be no view of justice discovered in the suffering, but, like Hauerwas, suggests that it may be that suffering is the key to bringing us to see and respond to the other.

Suffering gives us the possibility of overcoming the alienation and atomism experienced in Western society. The suffering of another enables us to be open to the real presence of the other, and leads to the development of responsibility for the other. The negativity and meaninglessness of the suffering, in effect, provides the real basis for contact with the other. Suffering grounds the ethical response, is the foundation of being responsible for the other. Once more there is the possible danger here of making suffering a means to an end. However, Levinas's point is that suffering is an inevitable and profound part of our lives and that compassion and empathy are the only way of making sense of it.

Van Hooft (1998) concludes:

> The challenge of postmodern authenticity is to sever the link between suffering and justice. It is to accept the blindness of fate and the inevitability of bad luck. It is to refuse the false consolations of theodicies or metaphysical theories which make suffering positive. (p19)

The conceptual understanding of theodicies can never of themselves begin to provide genuinely spiritual meaning for those who are experiencing suffering. Not only are they partial, in the sense that they are one of many different views, they are also generalized and purely cognitive. In order to discover meaning in suffering it has to be particular and has to engage the affective and somatic dimensions.

This does not mean that the conversation about justice ends here. Rather, it moves from the big question 'Why me?' across to the relationships of the sufferer, and the justice in them. Make no mistake, those who experience suffering do ask the kind of questions that the grand philosophers asked about fairness, but they only get an answer when they begin to look at themselves and their experience, and their responsibility within it. This seems to involve three things, transcendence, awareness and justice in relationships.

Transcendence

Spirituality can help one to transcend suffering. Whatever the cause, to simply survive in that situation demands locking into a higher sense of identity. This is exemplified by Campbell's (1995) example of the hostage Terry Waite. Waite transcended the effects of his long suffering through holding on to and developing the world of spiritual meaning – partly through repeated articulation of narrative, and partly through rehearsal of the meaning rituals relevant to his community of meaning. In all his isolation and deprivation, Terry Waite repeated the words of the Anglican Eucharist which he knew by heart, thus holding on to his life-meaning – church community, friends, spiritual ritual, and God – and thus his humanity, his human identity. The issue of justice became in this case secondary to survival.

Campbell suggests that how we deal with suffering in this light is, 'a product of our broader conception of how human life ought to be' (p.29). Yet it is more than simply a conception. It is also a product of the awareness of the spiritual environment within which such a conception is embodied. Such a conception involves cognitive, affective and somatic awareness of the self and the other, including the illness and the suffering itself. At the core of any understanding of health and suffering is how 'the self retains its dignity and worth' in the face of pain, disability, and death, three things that we all experience at some point in our lives (p.42).

There is a sense in which dignity itself involves justice. It is about doing justice to oneself, more than accepting, more than letting go. Like so many 'big' concepts dignity has been given a range of very different shades of meaning. Dignity broadly refers to honour and worth, the sense of being held in esteem. Maintenance of dignity is a function of a relationship that develops mutuality and enables the person to develop awareness of her relational network and her purpose in it. Terry Waite was able to simply reflect on his relationship networks. Others have to work through and make sense of these to affirm their own dignity. Dignity in other words is not something that is simply 'given', but rather emerges from a relationship, and is worked out in each situation.

Awareness

Spirituality in the midst of justice seems to increase a sense of environmental awareness. For example, Pat was diagnosed with a motor neurone disease. She eventually reached a stage where she was only able to move her head and her shoulders, and all she could do was to sit and look out of the window.

> I can see from my window at least fifteen big trees, and I used to think that would be boring. But after a while you can see the differences. One tree has a wasps nest in it, one has little flowers, one has a twisted trunk, and so on. But the amazing differences are the colours. I did not realize that there are so many different greens. It's not just one mass of green leaves along fifteen trees, it's a kaleidoscope of green. Then when the sun or the rain strikes they change again: trees that stand still yet are always changing.

In the midst of the experience of suffering there can be not just the transcendence of the experience but a transcendence that enables increased awareness of the self and of the environment, social and physical, and of different levels of meaning. This is precisely why Hugo Gryn could speak of finding his God the more he experienced the suffering of Auschwitz.

Building justice

The issue of justice in all this is not lost but actually is more sharply focused. It moves away from big issues of justice and fairness, 'Why me?' and 'How can this happen to me?' to immediate relationships and how justice is lived out in these. Justice in this context is worked out in terms of creative response. At one level this is about looking at significant relationships and working out what is needed. Patients who are dying often focus on fractured relationships. Pat, the person with motor neurone disease, wanted to resolve the desertion of her by her mother in her teenage years. Such a resolution was not a simple reconciliation. She still had a strong sense of anger about it, and above all wanted to communicate that anger to her, and hear her response. The relationship then had to be truthful. In effect Pat was working out the goal of justice for herself. It meant a meeting and a confronting of her mother with the truth, and a sharing of anger. What might happen from there would depend upon the response of her mother. When the meeting did occur there was a hard edge it. It involved a real condemnation of her mother's action. Her mother's experience of this was that she felt that she had been found guilty, like a prisoner at the dock. Her response of contrition, which was not immediate, led Pat to offer friendship – not the return of a mother/daughter relationship, but a relationship whose moral meaning needed to be worked through. Peace in all this demanded truth, the acknowledgement and validation of feelings of anger on the part of Pat and guilt on the part of her mother, and a working out of what the relationship might now mean. Forgiveness was not the goal of the process, and might not even have been possible. Equally, other options might have included calling the other to account more publicly. Forgiveness, Smedes (1998) argues, is really about accepting the humanity of the other, and this is built in the context of the truth in relationship.

This dynamic picks up something of the richness of the concept of *shalom*. *Shalom* is a Hebrew word meaning peace but includes a sense of wholeness, alongside a sense of justice (sometimes even victory). But as the concept matured over time it even took on a transformative meaning. In Hebrew prophecy this moved from peace between nations to a time when God will bring everything together as new creation. The peaceful creative transformation is summed up in the lines of Isaiah, the vision of sword beaten into ploughshares and spears into pruning hooks when:

Nation shall not lift up sword against nation,
Neither shall they learn war anymore

(Isaiah 2:4, Authorized version)

For Pat her creative and transformative response to suffering was to take the decision to be confirmed into the Christian church This led to a remarkable confirmation service in her home with friends and family gathered together and visibly affected by her courage and strong sense of peace.

At the base of this is the agapeic dynamic. How love and justice relate has been the focus of much discussion (Outka 1972; Woodhead 1992). In the context of care this *agape* ensures that peace and justice remain together, thus inevitably influencing the meaning of justice, such that it includes restorative justice. Perhaps more importantly the dynamic of *agape* means that the person is responsible for working out what justice means in his or her situation. Importantly, this means that forgiveness and reconciliation are not forced, but emerge, if they do, from the creative response.

As Lambourne (2004) notes, this could involve many different kinds and combinations of justice, including:

- *Retributive justice.* This is about settling accounts. For those who have suffered childhood abuse this may be the right road.

- *Restitutive justice.* This involves recovery of losses, compensations for pain.

- *Restorative justice.* This is restoring or healing relationships between conflicting parties.

- *Social justice.* In this, parties are given what they need to achieve social equality or resolution.

- *Distributive justice.* This is a fair distribution of goods according to need.

The important point in all this is that justice is focused in relationship, not in codes or rules. Furthermore, justice comes to life when we take responsibility for it.

Alan, a middle manager in a large corporation, suffering from stress, was referred to a counsellor. As the therapy progressed it became clear that he was the victim of oppression and injustice. His Chief Executive Officer (CEO) constantly fed too much work down to Alan, with the result that he regularly worked over the weekend. As Alan reflected on this he became more aware not simply of his stress, but of the stress that was being suffered by the dozen people who worked for him. Sure enough they too were working over weekends to hit deadlines on a regular basis.

Alan gradually became aware then that he was not only a victim of injustice but that he was also the cause of injustice to his staff. All the office and beyond knew what was happening, and many of his staff were receiving counselling. Only when he too became aware of this did justice become something that he felt he had to take responsibility for. This had been a major emotional blow to Alan, partly because he felt he was the victim, and partly because he prided himself as having a strong sense of justice. This meant that he had to critique what he meant by justice. In turn this led to a radical transformation of his relationship to his CEO and his staff.

This brings us back to the development of virtues. In this case the Aristotelian virtue of justice had to be developed by Alan. Often the concept of justice is seen as something elevated, a big idea applying to big situations. Worse still, it is seen by some as an abstract concept. Alan's case shows that justice, and responsibility for justice, is at the heart of everyday creative responses, and that justice demands holistic engagement, and individual acceptance of responsibility.

Freedom

The pursuit of justice in caring also relates closely to the development of freedom. Campbell (1995) characterizes spirituality as freedom, and there is no doubt that in addressing the spiritual dimension of ethics one of the outcomes is a complex and holistic freedom. This is not freedom in a limited sense of autonomy (either freedom of choice or freedom from coercion) but something far richer and complex:

- *Freedom from the tyranny of shame and sin.* As Vanier (1999) notes, this is a freedom based in truth which means that the person no longer has to expend energy on the protection of the false self, and is no longer dominated by a narrative of shame. Central to such freedom is the development of empathy and the capacity to transcend the self.

- *Freedom based in the truth of the situation.* This enables the person to accept what is, the reality of the situation that cannot be changed. This is the freedom of empathy, to live with ambiguities, and not having to resolve them, the freedom to be the self in spite of limitations, pain and suffering.

- *Freedom to belong.* Many who approach care services feel they are consigned to the margins of community. They do not feel they have permission to belong. *Agape* brings the freedom to trust, to know that one belongs, even if this begins in a community that is either very different or temporary.

- *Freedom to be responsible for the self and others.* Such responsibility is virtually impossible if it is seen only as a individualistic thing. Being part of a community means mutual responsibility and thus the possibility that the demands and claims of others be recognized, appreciated and responded to. This freedom is essentially social. In this the negotiation of responsibility frees the person up to share and thus take or let go of responsibility.

- *Freedom to work out purpose and make meaning.* This dynamic involves the articulation of the personal narrative, the development of the capacity to value and critique that narrative, an explicit and positive letting go the old moral world (whether its meaning was explicit or implicit) and creating and recreating moral meaning, through critical reflection on narratives and through practice.

- *Freedom to create.* Through hope and the creative imagination this freedom enables *shalom* to be achieved. Reality has been accepted, with its limitations and ambiguities, but reality is also created, transformed, through creative partnerships.

- *Freedom to learn.* Awareness of limitations and possibilities, the development of the capacity to accept and critique all enable the person to learn and so to change. With this is the freedom to take risks, not least the risk of disclosing the self, the risk of trusting an other, and the risk of being faithful to the other, waiting for her response.

- At the heart of many of these dimensions of freedom is the *freedom to critique.* Because criticism is so often associated with personal attack many people find it difficult to give or take critique of their thoughts or actions.

Freedom in all this emerges through the development of virtues and a related commitment, purpose, agency and practice. Mustakova-Possardt (2004) suggests, from the perspective of education for a critical moral consciousness, that the development of moral motivation is tied to such learning. She sets out four dimensions of such motivation:

- *Moral identity.* This moves beyond identity rooted in moral conventions to the acceptance of a concern to do the right thing not simply based on self or even mutual interest.

- *Authority, responsibility and agency.* This involves the development of the critical discernment of external moral authority, with an expanding sense of moral responsibility and moral agency.

- *Relationships.* In this there is a development of empathy, relatedness and concerns with justice.

- *Meaning of life.* This dimension involves a broader framework from which to reflect on value. Motivation comes from having an appreciation of purpose and its social and moral meaning.

Authority

Alongside freedom must come the question of authority. Browning (2006) and Mustakova-Possardt (2004) both argue that the critical hermeneutic and moral development do not take one away from the community of meaning but rather help one to recognize the authority of that community. For all Tawney's (1964) stress on equality he too looks to the recognition of leadership. But what, given a learning model, would such authority look like?

I would suggest that it could not be simply conceptual or institutional authority, i.e. authority invested in orthodoxy or formal roles. The whole point of the critical hermeneutic is that both of these are tested. Authority then becomes relational, focused in exactly the embodied care that I have outlined. The criteria of authority then become:

- love expressed in social contract

- empathy, enabling the affective dimension of truth to be accessed

- *phronesis*, practical wisdom that automatically asks questions of purpose

- integrity, enabling a relational authority that is transparent and which enables learning at community and individual level.

Such an authority can learn, change and still remain consistent, precisely because it does not place identity exclusively in an institution or concept. Identity, of course, also involves history and thus requires institutions and narratives to resource and articulate that history and the accumulated wisdom. They, and the practice of interpreting them, remain embodiments of the criteria of authority. This steers a path between authoritarianism and utopianism (Williams 2005).

Grace

At the heart of such authority is grace. This is not grace as 'a semi-material infused substance' (Schwobel 2000, p.278). It is rather the free gift of *agape*. The fact that the gift is genuinely free means that it brings with it no attempt to control. At the same time the gift has to be accepted freely, with no attempt on the part of the recipient to control it. This means that anyone giving care should not assume that change will occur or attempt to manipulate change. Care can only offer the care and enable the challenge. Assessing outcomes then becomes a matter of dialogue, not least in the negotiation of responsibilities.

The idea of grace extends to gracefulness, the image of the person who is co-ordinated – integrating the cognitive, affective, somatic and social. Grace then enables, and emerges from the agapeic relationship, with timing and awareness arising from empathy.

Enabling this graceful change, this constant creation and recreation of moral and spiritual meaning is what Vanier (1999) refers to as the 'accompanier' (p.128). There is a need for an other or more than one other, who can enable the person to develop empathy. These represent and are part of the community of care. Part of the image here is of the companion who joins the person for some part of their spiritual and moral journey, helping her to make that journey. Equally interesting is the image of the musical accompanist. The accompanist provides the support for the singer to express her narrative. It is not simply the repetition of notes. Rather does the accompanist enter real dialogue with the singer echoing phrases of the song, providing harmonies that deepen the meaning of the song, often working through dissonance, and together with the singer to create the affective and cognitive meaning of the words. It is this dialogue and reflection which enables the change that maintains the continuity of personal identity and the development of meaning.

The land of Serendip

If the ethical response is part of the spiritual journey, of the person and the community, then it is essentially risky. We may make the journey with a spiritual map, but we are still discovering what lies ahead, and developing that map. Lederach (2005) suggests this makes work with the moral imagination essentially serendipitous. He reminds us that the word first came from Horace Walpole's letter of 1754 in which he refers to a Persian tale of the three Princes from Serendip. As they travelled 'they were always making discoveries, by accident and sagacity of things they were not in quest of' (quoted in Lederach 2005, p.114). This suggests the essential obliquity of ethics which takes spirituality seriously. What one learns about others, oneself, one's community, one's responsibility and the possibilities of creative response cannot be charted in a straight line, from doctrine to outcome. We are likely to be surprised by where that journey take us and what we find along the way. In the same way the virtues developed are not explicitly aimed for. They arise out of a journey charted by *agape*.

The domain of spirituality

Of course, the spiritual cartographers of the past were mostly theologians or occasional philosophers. They have now been joined by psychologists, educationalists, and those in the care professions. In many cases they do not import spiritual and moral ideas but rather validate, and amplify the ones that are already there, expressed by the patient or client. All of this reminds us that no group has exclusive rights on the moral imagination and its spiritual dynamic, precisely because at its centre is empathic transcendence that takes us beyond the self and the group, and which engages the plurality within the group (Lederach 2005).

This presents a major challenge to religious writers such as Hauerwas (1986), Pattison (2001), and Milbank (1990). Each of these, in different ways, stresses the primary importance of articulating the Christian narrative, about the spirit with a capital 'S'. From the same position one can hear of the need to speak the word of prophecy to the 'secular' world, as if indeed this is the word of prophecy. This puts me in mind of a university chaplains' conference where one eager chaplain sprang to his feet and cried out 'I have found the role of the chaplain'. He continued 'It is to be the prophet to the university, to speak out against the false targets and the injustice'. For a moment there was a corporate intake of breath. Yes, perhaps he had found our real identity and purpose. Then another chaplain stood up and asked him, 'and how does our prophecy relate to the other prophets on campus, the student union, the staff who blow the whistle, the governors who seek justice in committee, the vice-chancellor who wants to develop a caring ethos, the counsellor who stands up for student rights, the campus doctor…' Prophecy, in the sense of standing out against injustice, is not the function of one group, but rather of the dialogue and working together of many. This is precisely the creative and transformative dynamic of the moral imagination. Sometimes, one group may stand out in order to speak to the others, but the same group at another time may have to hear the prophetic word as applied to them. It was precisely the judges, for instance, who enabled dialogue and critique of the church's position in the conjoined twins case. The Christian church, which has caused so much violence as well as building so much peace should above all recognize the need for humility and empathy in the exercise of prophecy. This contrasts sharply with the idea that the Christian church should try to 'out-narrate' other philosophies.

As noted above, the narrative is in fact the vehicle of spirituality and as such develops reflection, dialogue, empathy, transcendence, responsibility and response. Such a dialogue enables mutual revelation and mutual challenge, confirming and developing identity, and revealing what is possible. No religion has anything to fear from such a dialogue, least of all loss of identity. This would involve religions recognizing and engaging with the spirituality of the other. Accepting this generic view of spirituality, far from diluting the narrative of religions actually enables a mutual dialogue that enables others to understand the nature of faith, and with that the particular nature of particular faith narratives. In this sense inter-faith dialogue extends well beyond different religions.

Conclusions

In this book I have tried to show how spirituality is intimately connected to ethics. Moral responsibility lies at the base of spirituality. Ethical decisions do not emerge seamlessly from set cognitive doctrines but require a wrestling with tradition and plurality that is there in the life of the patient and his or her communities. This is not a simple matter of something called 'ethics' wrestling with something called 'spirituality'. It involves doctrines, traditions, narratives, codes – all of which are founded and sustained in relationships, be they family, work, or church. In these, ethics becomes connected with the existential realities of faith, hope, and purpose. Hence, wrestling demands an emotional as well as cognitive engagement, enabling reflection that genuinely tests and develops identity. Such identity is confirmed and further developed through commitment to people and practice. Indeed, spirituality can only take wing in practice – real projects (Lederach 2005). Such practice requires that responsibility is shared through effective negotiation.

From the moral imperative of responsibility for the other, spirituality then moves into creative, transformative response, and resolution. I have noted that this is a development of virtue ethics. It is also a development of the feminist ethics of care (Koehn 1998). Like them, it stresses relationality, and underlying concepts of care, empathy and trust.

However, it moves further into doctrinal and existential meaning, not least in faith and hope, and into the embodiment of that meaning in creative response. However, just as important as locating this approach in the wider ethical scene is to be aware that persons who have to make significant decisions in the areas of care, clients and professional's alike, can and do (when given the space to reflect and dialogue) work through exactly the moral and spiritual issues that these different ethical schools wrestle with, even to the extent of developing value and virtue vocabulary. I hope, in providing several actual cases, to have demonstrated these issues are for ordinary people, not just philosophers or theologians, and that given space in the community of care they also can contribute creative responses that can further develop moral and spiritual meaning.

In all this, spirituality cannot be seen simply as individualistic, with the person choosing to take what they want from 'religious experience'. It is about making sense of and responding to the communities of which we are a part, from local to global, from family to environment. It is precisely because of this that spirituality cannot be summed up in terms of rights language. Yes, everyone has the right to work through their own spirituality, but precisely because it is embedded in moral responsibility, and is a part of and responsive to the person's social and physical environment, it is relation- and not individual-centred. Hence, it requires learning and testing and commitment to the other. Hence, the spirituality and the values that emerge from it can never be simply about tolerating faith, but rather are to do with engaging and valuing it.

This translates into the caring community through the idea of covenant and shared responsibility. It is not the task of that community to solve problems for the patient or client, but to provide the environment in which they can make sense of their experience, not as something discrete or self contained, but rather something lived in relationship. It is still up to them to take responsibility for that reflection, and therefore their choice.

However good the community of care, the spiritual journey is never completed. By definition spirituality is an ongoing and holistic experience. However, in many cases the change that this approach offers is central to the therapeutic process, including cancer and palliative care (Robinson and Dodsworth 2002), MI, addictions, mental health (Swinton 2001), bereavement care, and also more chronic conditions.

The practical applications of this approach are straightforward:

1. Where there is a major ethical decision to be made, it is important to give those involved in making it space for underlying spirituality to be explored. The ethical situation involves far more than just a discrete decision.

2. Where there is life change signalled as part of therapy it is important to enable the patient to connect this to their existing beliefs and values. Without these connections, moral meaning and agency are hard to develop – and without that key ground for motivation is lost. All too often ethics books ignore this kind of case. However, the ethical dimension of such life change is quite as great as major ethical cases such as the conjoined twins. Any life change will involve change of values and behaviour, will affect many people beyond the patient, and need to involve a conscious working out of ethical values.

3. Where there is sign of spiritual tension, around purpose and life-meaning, and there is no obvious life-changing crisis involved it is important to give space to the patient or client to work through their story. It may be important for the patient or client to lock into spirituality as a coping mechanism, or to develop new meaning. There is within care the danger of medicalizing spirituality. Hence, many writers (see Robinson *et al.* 2003) refer to 'spiritual pain' or 'spiritual distress'. The danger then is to think of this pain or distress as a 'condition' that requires intervention or a problem that needs to be solved. In fact, for many, the apparent distress can be positive and potentially life-enhancing, needing not care in the form of service to alleviate the distress, but care in the form of being given space to wrestle with issues. Lederach (2005) suggests that conflict is an inevitable part of life and that dealing with it is part of a positive spiritual engagement. The responsibility for providing such space is that of the community of care, and not just of one specialist group. This means clarity about responsibility negotiation. In one cardiac care team, for instance, the lead surgeon decided that it was his role 'to remind patients of their mortality'. This meant showing them in a caring way how close they had been to death. The effect on the patient was usually intense, and space was provided for reflection by the rest of the team, sometimes with nurses, sometimes with chaplains or counsellors. Where teams are limited then they can point beyond the community of care to other places where such space can be found.

4. The community of care has to work continuously at reflecting on its meaning. This means working against teleopathy – be that obsession with targets or consumerism – and working positively to communicate its beliefs and values. Bauman continuously reminds us that rational planning without responsibility can lead to a breakdown of moral meaning that it is all too easy to miss.

5. The community of care can finally begin to enable the professional, patient or client to begin to make a difference in practice. The difference is first about how we see the world, in being able to see and acknowledge the stranger. From such awareness emerges the possibility of response to the other, and with that hope. From such hope emerges action that embodies the moral imagination, and so beings to transform all who are involved. It is the creation of new and creative community, not perfect, but founded on care, commitment and responsibility at individual and at community level. This is not about simple or easy solutions but rather action that always reflects on values and our awareness of the other, and that makes all the difference in the world.

References

Albin, T. (1988) 'Spirituality.' In S. Ferguson and D. Wright (eds) *New Dictionary of Theology*. Leicester: IVP.

Alcoholics Anonymous (1976) (3rd edn) New York: Alcoholics Anonymous World Services.

AACN (American Association of Colleges of Nursing) (1986) *Essentials of College and University Education for Nursing*. Washington: AACN.

Anon. (2006) 'Shelved Muhammad Opera to Return.' Available online at http://news.bbc.co.uk/1/hi/entertainment/6091624.stm (accessed 16 july 2007).

Aquinas (1981) *Summa Theologica*. New York: Resources for Christian Living.

Avis, P. (1989) *Eros and the Sacred*. London: SPCK.

Backhouse, S., Mckenna, J. and Robinson, S. (2007) *Motivation and Performance Enhancing Drugs*. New York: World Anti Drugs Agency.

Baggott, R. (1994) *Health and Health Care in Britain*. London: Palgrave Macmillan.

Baird, M. (2002) *On the Side of the Angels: Ethics and Post Holocaust Spirituality*. Leuven: Peeters.

Bakhtin, M. (1984) *Problems of Dostoevsky's Poetics*, tr. C. Emerson. Minneapolis: University of Minnesota Press.

Bakhtin, M.M. (1993) *Towards a Philosophy of the Act*. Houston: University of Texas Press.

Barker. E. (1992) *New Religious Movements*. London: HMSO.

Barnett, R. (1994) *The Idea of Higher Education*. Buckingham: Open University Press.

Baudrillard, J. (1983) *Simulations*. New York: Semiotext.

Bauman, Z. (1989) *Modernity and the Holocaust*. London: Polity.

Bauman, Z. (1993) *Postmodern Ethics*. Oxford: Blackwell.

Beauchamp, T. and Childress, T. (1994) *Principles of Biomedical Ethics* (4th edn) New York: Oxford University Press.

Beck, J. (1999) '"Spiritual and Moral Development" and Religious Education.' In A. Thatcher (ed.) (1999) *Spirituality and the Curriculum*. London: Cassell.

Beckett, C. and Maynard, A. (2005) *Values and Ethics in Social Work*. London: Sage.

Belenky, M. (1986) *Women's Ways of Knowing*. New York: Basic Books.

Bellamy, J. (1998) 'Spiritual Values in a Secular Age.' In M. Cobb and V. Renshaw (eds) *The Spiritual Challenge of Health Care*. London: Churchill.

Bender, T. (2005) 'From Academic Knowledge to Democratic Knowledge.' In S. Robinson and C. Katulushi *Values in Higher Education*. Cardiff: Aureus.

Benson, H. (1996) *Timeless Healing*. New York: Scribner.

Bernardi, L., Sleight, P., Bandinelli, G., Cencetti, S., Fatorini, L., Wdowczyc-Szulc, J. and Lagi, A. (2001) 'Effect of Rosary Prayer and Yoga Mantras on Autonomic Cardiovascular Rhythms: Comparative Study.' *British Medical Journal* 323, 922–9, 1446–9.

Berryman, J. (1985) 'Children's spirituality and religious language.' *British Journal of Religious Education* 7, 3, Summer.

Biggar, N. (1997) *Good Life*. London: SPCK.

Bilgrami, A. (1992) 'What is a Muslim? Fundamental commitment and cultural identity.' *Critical Inquiry 18*, 4, 821–842.

Billings, A. (1992) 'Pastors or Counsellors?' *Contact 108*, 2, 3–9.

Boyd, J. (1995) 'The soul as seen through evangelical eyes, part 1.' *Journal of Psychology and Theology 25*, 3, 151–160.

Bradshaw, A. (1994) *Lighting the Lamp; The Spiritual Dimension of Nursing Care*. London: Scutari Press.

Breuggemann, W. (1984) *The Message of the Psalms*. Minneapolis: Augsburg.

Brueggemann, W. (1997) *Theology of the Old Testament*. Nashville: Abingdon.

Bridges, W. (1980) *Transitions: Making Sense of Life's Changes*. Reading Mass.: Addison Wesley.

Browning, D. (1983) *Religious Ethics and Pastoral Care*. Philadelphia: Fortress.

Browning, D. (2006) *Christian Ethics and Moral Psychologies*. Grand Rapids: Eerdmans.

Brummer, V. (1993) *The Model of Love*. Cambridge: Cambridge University Press.

Buber, M. (1937) *I and Thou*. Edinburgh: T. and T. Clark.

Burleigh, M. (2000) *The Third Reich: A New History*. London: Macmillan.

Campbell, A. (1984) *Moderated Love: A Theology of Professional Care*. London: SPCK.

Campbell, A. (1995) *Health As Liberation*. Cleveland: The Pilgrim Press.

Campbell, A. (2003) 'The virtues (and vices) of the four principles.' *Journal of Medical Ethics 29*, 292–296.

Campbell, A. and Swift, T. (2002) 'What does it mean to be a virtuous patient?' *Scottish Journal of Health Care Chaplaincy 5*, 29–35.

Canda, E. (1989) 'Religious content in social work education.' *Journal of Social Work Education 30*, 1, 38–45.

Cantwell Smith, W. (1998) *Faith and Belief: The Difference Between Them*. Princeton N.J.: Princeton University Press.

Carter, R. (1985) 'A taxonomy of objectives for professional education.' *Studies in Higher Education 10*, 2, 135–149.

Cashman, H. (1992) *Christianity and Child Sexual Abuse*. London: SPCK.

Cho, F. (2005) 'Ritual.' In W. Schweiker (ed.) *The Blackwell Companion to Religious Ethics*. Oxford: Blackwell.

Church of England, Anglican Bishops (1996) *Issues in Human Sexuality*. London: Church House.

Clinebell, H. (1990) 'Alcohol Abuse, Addiction and Therapy.' In R. Hunter (ed.) *Dictionary of Pastoral Care and Counseling*. Nashville: Abingdon Press.

Cole, B. and Pargament, K. (2003) 'Spiritual Surrender: A Paradoxical Path to Control.' In W. Miller (ed.) *Integrating Spirituality into Treatment*. Washington: American Psychological Association.

Connor, S. (1989) *The Post Modern Culture*. Oxford: Blackwell.

Connors, G., Toscova, R. and Tonigan, J. (2003) 'Serenity.' In W. Miller (ed.) *Integrating Spirituality into Treatment*. Washington: American Psychological Association.

Cooper, B. (2002) *Teachers as Moral Models? – The Role of Empathy on Relationships Between Pupils and Their Teachers*. Unpublished PhD Thesis, University of Leeds.

Damasio, A. (1994) *Descartes' Error*. New York: Putnam.

DOH (Department of Health) (2001) *Your Guide to the NHS*. London: Department of Health.

Department of Health and King's Fund (2006) *Improving the Patient Experience – Celebrating Achievement: Enhancing the Healing Environment Programme*. London: TSO.

Doyle, D. (1992) 'Have we looked beyond the physical and psychosocial?' *Journal of Pain Management 7,5*, 301–311.

Edwards, D. (1999) *After Death?* London: Cassell.

Elder, L. (2000) 'Why some Jehovah's Witnesses accept blood and conscientiously reject official Watchtower Society blood policy.' *Journal of Medical Ethics 26*: 375–380.

Ellison, C. (1983) 'Spiritual well-being: conceptualization and measurement.' *Journal of Psychology and Theology 11*, 4, 11–21.

Employment Equality (Religion and Belief) Regulations SI (2003) No. 1660, London: HMSO.

Erikson, E. (1959) *Identity and the Life Cycle*. New York: International Universities Press.

Erikson, R. (1987) 'The psychology of self-esteem: promise or peril?' *Pastoral Psychology 35*, 3, Spring, 163–171.

Fasching, D. (1992) *Narrative Theology after Auschwitz*. Minneapolis: Fortress Press.

Fasching, D. and Dechant, D. (2001) *Comparative Religious Ethics*. Oxford: Blackwell.

Fiddes, P. (2000) *Participating in God*. London: Darton, Longman and Todd.

Finch, J. and Mason, J. (1993) *Negotiating Family Responsibilities*. London: Routledge.

Fleischacker, S. (1994) *The Ethics of Culture*. Ithaca: Cornell University Press.

Florman, S. (1976) *The Existential Pleasures of Engineering*. New York: St. Martins.

Fontana, D. (2003) *Psychology, Religion and Spirituality*. Oxford: Blackwell.

Ford, D. (1999) *Self and Salvation*. Cambridge: Cambridge University Press.

Fowler, J. (1990) 'Faith/Belief.' In R. Hunter (ed.) *Dictionary of Pastoral Care and Counseling*. Nashville: Abingdon.

Fowler, J. (1996) *Faithful Change*. Nashville: Abingdon.

Frankena, W. (1986) 'The Relations of Morality and Religion.' In J. McQuarrie (ed.) *A New Dictionary of Christian Ethics*. London: SCM.

Freeman, M. (1993) *Rewriting the Self*. London: Routledge.

Gadamer, H-G. (1982) *Truth and Method*. New York: Crossroad.

Gaita, R. (2000) *A Common Humanity*. London: Routledge.

Gamwell, F. (2005) 'Norms, Values and Metaphysics.' In W. Schweiker (ed.) *The Blackwell Companion to Religious Ethics*. Oxford: Blackwell.

Gibran, K. (1995) *The Prophet*. London: Penguin.

Gillman, P. 'Left to die at the top of the world.' The Sunday Times Magazine, 24 September 2006.

Gillon, R. (2000) 'Refusal of potentially life-saving blood transfusions by Jehovah's Witnesses: should doctors explain that not all JWs think it's religiously required?' *Journal of Medical Ethics 26*, 299–301.

Gillon, R. (2003) 'Four scenarios.' *Journal of Medical Ethics. 29*, 267–268.

Goddard, N. (1995) 'Spirituality as integrative energy.' *Journal of Advanced Nursing 22*, 808–815.

Goldstein, J. and Kornfield, J. (1987) *Seeking the Heart of Wisdom*. Boston: Shambhala.

Grelle, B. (2005) 'Culture and Moral Pluralism.' In W. Schweiker (ed.) *The Blackwell Companion to Religious Ethics*. Oxford: Blackwell.

Griffin, A. (1983) 'A philosophical analysis of caring in nursing.' *Journal of Advanced Nursing 8*, 289–295.

Gryn, H. (2000) *Chasing Shadows*. London: Viking.

Gutiérrez, G. (1988) *A Theology of Liberation*. New York: Orbis Books.

Habermas, J. (1992) *Moral Consciousness and Communicative Action*. London: Polity.

Halmos, P. (1966) *Faith of the Counsellor*. London: Constable.

Halstead, J. (2005) 'Islam, homophobia and education; a reply to Michael Merry.' *Journal of Moral Education 34*, 1, March, 37–42.

Hamer, S. and Collinson, G. (1999) *Achieving Evidence-Based Practice*. London: Baillière Tindall.

Hart, K. (2004) *Postmodernism*. Oxford: One World.

Hauerwas, S. (1981) *Vision and Virtue*. Notre Dame: University of Notre Dame Press.

Hauerwas, S. (1984) *The Peaceable Kingdom*. London: SCM.

Hauerwas, S. (1986) *Suffering Presence*. Notre Dame: University of Notre Dame Press.

Hauerwas, S. and Wells, S. (eds) (2004) *The Blackwell Companion to Christian Ethics*. Oxford: Blackwell.

Hawkins, P. (1991) 'The spiritual dimension of the learning organisation.' *Management, Education and Development 22*, 3, 172–187.

Haydon, G. (2006) 'On the duty of educating respect: a response to Robin Barrow.' *Journal of Moral Education 35*, 1, March, 19–32.

Helminiak, D. (1998) 'Sexuality and spirituality: a humanist account' *Pastoral Psychology 47*, 2, 119–126.

Hiatt, J. (1986) 'Spirituality, medicine and healing.' *Southern Medical Journal 79*, 6, 736–43.

Highfield, M. (1992) 'Spiritual health of oncology patients. Nurse and patient perspectives.' *Cancer Nursing 15*, 1, 1–8.

Hoffman, M. (2000) *Empathy and Moral Development: Implications for Caring and Justice.* Cambridge: Cambridge University Press.

Holloway, R. (1999) *Godless Morality.* Edinburgh: Canongate.

Hull, J. (1991) *What Prevents Christian Adults from Learning.* Philadelphia: Trinity Press.

Jackson, T. (2003) *The Priority of Love.* Princeton: Princeton University Press.

John Paul II (1995) *Evangelium Vitae.* Rome: Vatican.

Johnson, J. (1991) 'Learning to Live Again: The Process of Adjustment Following a Heart Attack.' In J. Morse and J. Johnson (eds) *The Illness Experience: Dimensions of Suffering.* London: Sage.

Joseph, M. (1998) 'The effect of strong religious concepts on coping with stress.' *Stress Medicine 14*, 219–224.

Jungel, E. (1983) *God as the Mystery of the World*, tr. D. Guder. Edinburgh: T. and T. Clark.

Kaufman, G. (1980) *Shame: The Power of Caring.* Washington: Schenkman.

Kelly, T. (1990) *A New Imagining: Towards and Australian Spirituality.* Melbourne: Collins Dove.

Kendrick, K. and Robinson, S. (2002) *Their Rights: Advance Directives and Living Wills.* London: Age Concern.

Kierkegaard, S. (1946) *Works of Love.* Princeton: Princeton University Press.

King, M. and Dein, S. (1998) 'The spiritual variable in psychiatric research' *Psychological Medicine 28*, 1259–1262.

Koehn, D. (1998) *Rethinking Feminist Ethics.* London: Routledge.

Kohlberg, L. (1984) *Essays on Moral Development Vol. 2: The Psychology of Moral Development.* San Francisco: Harper and Row.

Kohut, H. (1982) 'Introspection, empathy and the semi circle of mental health.' *International Journal of Psychoanalysis 663.*

Kristjansson, K. (2004) 'Empathy, sympathy, justice and the child' *Journal of Moral Education 33*, 3, 291–306.

Lambourne, W. (2004) 'Post-Conflict Peacebuilding.' *Peace, Conflict and Development 4*, April, 1–24.

Laming, Lord H. (2003) *Report of an Inquiry into the Death of Victoria Climbié.* London: The Stationery Office.

Lapsley, D. and Navarez, D. (2006) 'Character Education.' In A. Renninger I. and Siegel (eds) *Handbook of Child Psychology.* New York: Wiley.

Lartey, E. (1997) *In Living Colour.* London: Cassell.

Lederach, J.P. (2005) *The Moral Imagination: The Art and Soul of Building Peace.* Oxford: Oxford University Press.

Lee, S. (2003) *Uneasy Ethics.* London: Pimlico.

Lester, A. (1995) *Hope in Pastoral Care and Counselling.* Louisville: John Knox Press.

Levinas, E. (1988) 'Useless Suffering.' In R. Bernasconi and D. Wood (eds) *The Provocation of Levinas: Rethinking the Other.* London: Routledge.

Levinas, E. (1998) *Entre Nous: On Thinking-of-the-Other.* New York: Columbia University Press.

Levine, M. (1990) 'Nursing Ethics and the Ethical Nurse.' In J. Thompson and H. Thompson (eds) *Professional Ethics in Nursing.* Malabor: Krieger.

Lovin, R. (2005) 'Moral Theories.' In W. Schweiker (ed.) *The Blackwell Companion to Religious Ethics.* Oxford: Blackwell.

Lyotard, J-F. (1979) *The Postmodern Condition.* Manchester: Manchester University Press.

Margulies, A. (1989) *The Empathic Imagination.* New York: W.W. Norton.

Markham, I. (1994) *Plurality and Christian Ethics.* Cambridge: Cambridge University Press.

Marlatt, G. and Kristeller, J. (2003) 'Mindfulness and Meditation.' In W. Miller (ed.) *Integrating Spirituality into Treatment.* Washington: American Psychological Association.

May, W. (1987) 'Code and Covenant or Philanthropy?' In S. Lammers and A. Verhey (eds) *On Moral Medicine.* Grand Rapids: Eerdmans.

May, W. (1994) 'The Virtues in the Professional Setting.' In J. Soskice (ed.) *Medicine and Moral Reasoning.* Cambridge: Cambridge University Press.

Mayer, J. (1992) 'Wholly responsible for a part, or partly responsible for the whole? The concept of spiritual care in nursing.' *Second Opinion* 26–55.

Mbiti, J. (1990) *African Religions and Philosophy.* London: Heinemann.

McCullough, M. and Larson, D. (2003) 'Prayer.' In W. Miller (ed.) *Integrating Spirituality into Treatment.* Washington: American Psychological Association.

McFadyen, A. (1990) *The Call to Personhood.* Cambridge: Cambridge University Press.

McFague, S. (1997) *Super, Natural Christians.* London: SCM.

McIntyre, A. (1981) *After Virtue.* London: Duckworth.

McIntyre, A. (1999) *Dependent Rational Animals.* London: Duckworth.

McLeish, T. (2005) 'Values and Scientific Research.' In S. Robinson and C. Katulushi *Values in Higher Education.* Cardiff: Aureus.

Meeks, W. (1989) *God the Economist: the Doctrine of God and the Political Economy.* Minneapolis: Fortress.

Meeks, W. (1993) *The Origin of Christian Morality.* New Haven: Yale University Press.

Meilander, G. (1984) *The Theory and Practice of Virtue.* Notre Dame: Notre Dame Press.

Merry, M. (2005) 'Should educators accommodate intolerance?' *Journal of Moral Education 34*,1, March, 19–36.

Michel, T. (2005) 'The Ethics of Pardon and Peace.' In I. Markham and I. Ozdemir (eds) *Globalization, Ethics and Islam.* Aldershot: Ashgate.

Milbank, J. (1990) *Theology and Secular Reason: Beyond Secular Reason.* Oxford: Blackwells.

Milgram, S. (2005) *Obedience to Authority.* New York: Pinter and Martin.

Miller, W. (ed.) (2003) *Integrating Spirituality into Treatment.* Washington: American Psychological Association.

Minow, M. (2006) 'What the rule of law should mean in civics education.' *Journal of Moral Education 35*, 2, June, 137–162.

Muramoto, O. (1998) 'Bioethics of the refusal of blood by Jehovah's Witnesses.' *Journal of Medical Ethics 24*, 223–230.

Murdoch, I. (1972) *The Sovereignty of the Good.* New York: Schucker.

Murdoch, I. (1993) *Metaphysics as a Guide to Morals.* London: Vintage.

Mustakova-Possardt, E. (2004) 'Education for Critical Moral Consciousness.' *Journal of Moral Education 33*, September, pp.245–70.

Nelson, J. (1978) *Embodiment.* Minneapolis: Augsburg.

Nouwen, H. (1994) *The Wounded Healer.* London: Darton, Longman and Todd.

Nussbaum, M. (1999) 'Human Functioning and Social Justice.' In C. Koggel (ed.) *Moral Issues in Global Perspective.* New York: Broadview Press.

Nygren, A. (1932) *Agape and Eros.* Philadelphia: Westminster Press.

O'Brien, M. (1998) *Spirituality in Nursing.* Boston: Jones and Bartlett.

O'Neil, F. (2006) *Assessing the Successes and Impact of the Ward Housekeeper Role.* The Centre for the Development of Healthcare Policy and Practice, University of Leeds.

O'Neill, O. (2002) *Autonomy and Trust in Bioethics.* Cambridge: Cambridge University Press.

Oldnall, A. (1996) 'A critical analysis of nursing: meeting the spiritual needs of the patient.' *Journal of Advanced Nursing 23*, 138–144.

Oppenheimer, H. (1983) *The Hope of Happiness.* London; SCM.

Otto, R. (1923) *The Idea of the Holy.* Oxford: Oxford University Press.

Outka, G. (1972) *Agape: An Ethical Analysis.* New Haven: Yale University Press.

Papadopoulos, I. (1999) 'Spirituality and holistic caring: and exploration of the literature.' *Implicit Religion 2*, 2, Nov.

Parks, S. (1992) 'Fowler Evaluated.' In J. Astley and L. Francis (eds) *Christian Perspectives on Faith Development*. Leominster: Gracewing.

Parry, J. (1988) 'Physical Education as Olympic Education.' *European Physical Education Review 4*, 2, 1–14.

Parry, J., Robinson, S. Nesti, M. and Watson, N. (2007) *Spirituality and Sport*. London: Routledge.

Pattison, S. (2001) 'Dumbing down the Spirit.' In H. Orchard (ed.) *Spirituality in Health Care Contexts*. London: Jessica Kingsley Publishers.

Perry, M. (1992) *Gods Within*. London: SPCK.

Perry, M. (1995) 'Idealism and Drift.' In J. Watt (ed.) *The Church, Medicine and the New Age*. London: The Churches' Council for Health and Healing.

Piaget, J. (1965) *The Moral Judgement of the Child*. New York: Free Press.

Pipher, M. (1996) *The Shelter of Each Other: Rebuilding our Families*. New York: Ballantine.

Plato, tr. G. Grube (2002) *Five Dialogues*. London: Hackett Publishing.

Rae, D. (1981) *Equalities*. Cambridge, Mass.: Harvard University Press.

Reader, J. (1997) *Beyond All Reason*. Cardiff: Aureus.

Reed, P. (1987) 'Spirituality and well-being in terminally ill hospitalised adults.' *Research in Nursing and Health 10*, 5, 335–344.

Reed, P. (1998) 'The re-enchantment of health care: a paradigm of spirituality.' In H. Reid (2006) 'Olympic Sport and its Lessons for Peace' *Journal of the Philosophy of Sport 33*, 205–214.

Reid, H. (2006) 'Olympic Sport and Its Lessons of Peace.' *Journal of the Philosophy of Sport 33*, 205–214.

Reynolds, F. and Schofer, J. (2005) 'Cosmology.' In W. Schweiker (ed.) *The Blackwell Companion to Religious Ethics*. Oxford: Blackwell.

Ricoeur, P. (1982) *Hermeneutics and the Human Sciences*. Cambridge: Cambridge University Press.

Ricoeur, P. (1992) *Oneself as Another*. Chicago: Chicago University Press.

Richards, P. and Bergin, A. (1997) *A Spiritual Strategy for Counseling and Psychotherapy*. Washington: American Psychological Association.

Richards, P., Rector, J. and Tjeltveit, A. (2003) 'Values, Spirituality and Psychotherapy.' In W. Miller (ed.) *Integrating Spirituality into Treatment*. Washington: American Psychological Association.

Robinson, S. (1998) 'Helping the Hopeless.' *Contact 127*, 3–11.

Robinson, S. (2001) *Agape, Moral Meaning and Pastoral Counselling*. Cardiff: Aureus.

Robinson, S. (2002) 'Nestlé, Baby Milk Substitute and International Marketing.' In C. Megone and S. Robinson (2002) *Case Histories and Business Ethics*. London: Routledge.

Robinson, S. (2004) *Ministry Among Students*. London, Canterbury: SCM.

Robinson, S. and Dixon, J.R. (1997) 'The professional engineer: virtues and learning.' *Science and Engineering Ethics 3*, 3, 339–348.

Robinson, S. and Dodsworth, P. (2002) 'Advancing Practice in Cancer Care Ethics.' In D. Clarke, J. Flanagan and K. Kendrick (eds) *Advancing Nursing Practice in Cancer and Palliative Care*. Basingstoke: Palgrave.

Robinson, S., Kendrick, K. and Brown, A. (2003) *Spirituality and the Practice of Healthcare*. Basingstoke: Palgrave.

Rogers, C. (1942) *Counseling and Psychotherapy*. London: Constable.

Rogers, C. (1983) *Freedom to Learn*. Columbus: Merrill.

Ruether, R.R. (1975) *New Women New Earth*. New York: Seabury Press.

Sanderson, C. and Linehan, M. (2003) 'Acceptance and Forgiveness.' In W. Miller (ed.) *Integrating Spirituality into Treatment*. Washington: American Psychological Association.

Schall, J. (2007) *The Regensburg Lecture*. Washington: St Augustine's Press.

Schrage, W. (1988) *The Ethics of the New Testament.* Edinburgh: T. and T. Clark.

Schlauch, E. (1990) 'Empathy as the essence of pastoral psychotherapy.' *The Journal of Pastoral Care,* Spring, *XLIV,* 1, 3–17.

Schoen, D. (1983) *The Reflective Practitioner.* New York: Basic Books.

Schotroff, L. (1978) 'Non-violence and the Love of One's Enemies.' In R.H. Fuller (ed.) *Essays on the Love Commandment.* Minneapolis: Fortress.

Schwobel, C. (2000) 'Grace.' In A. Hastings (ed.) *Oxford Companion to Christian Thought.* Oxford: Oxford University Press.

Seedhouse, D. (2002) *Ethics: the Heart of Health Care.* London: Wiley.

Segal, Z., Williams, J. and Teasdale, J. (2002) *Mindfulness-based Cognitive Therapy for Depression: A New Approach to Preventing Relapse.* New York: Guilford Publications.

Selby, P. (1983) *Liberating God.* London: SPCK.

Sidorkin, A. (1999) *Beyond Discourse: Education, the Self and Dialogue.* Albany: State University of New York Press.

Sims, A. (1994) 'Psyche-spirit as well as mind?' *British Journal of Psychiatry 165,* 441–446.

Smail, D. (1984) *Illusion and Reality: The Meaning of Anxiety.* London: J.M. Dent.

Smedes, L. (1998) 'Stations on the Journey from Forgiveness to Hope.' In E. Worthington Jr. *Dimensions of Forgiveness.* Philadelphia: Templeton Foundation.

Snyder, C. (2000) 'The past and possible futures of hope.' *Journal of Social and Clinical Psychology 19,* 1, Spring 2000, 11–28.

Solomon, R. (1992) *Ethics and Excellence.* Oxford: Oxford University Press.

Spohn, W. (1997) 'Spirituality and ethics: Exploring the connections' *Theological Studies 58,* 109–122.

Spohn, W. (2003) 'Spirituality and Its Discontents.' *Journal of Religious Ethics 32,* 2, 253–276.

Stern, D. (1985) *The Interpersonal World of the Infant.* New York: Basic Books.

Sternberg, E. (2000) *Just Business.* Oxford: Oxford University Press.

Swift, T., Ashcroft, A., Tadd, W., Campbell, A. and Dieppe, P. (2002) 'Living well through chronic illness: the relevance of virtue theory to patients with chronic osteoarthritis,' *Arthritis Care and Research 47,* 5, 474–478.

Swinton, J. (2001) *Spirituality and Mental Health Care.* London: Jessica Kingsley Publishers.

Tangney J. (2000) 'Humility: Theoretical perspectives, empirical findings and directions for future research.' *Journal of Social and Clinical Psychology 19,* 1, Spring, 70–82.

Tawney, R.H. (1964) *Equality.* London: Allen and Unwin.

Tawney, R.H. (1972) *The Commonplace Book.* Cambridge: Cambridge University Press.

Taylor, C. (1983) *Human Agency and Language.* Cambridge: Cambridge University Press.

Taylor, C. (1989) *Sources of the Self.* Cambridge: Cambridge University Press.

Taylor, C. (1996) 'Iris Murdoch and Moral Philosophy.' In M. Antonaccio and W. Schweiker (eds) *Iris Murdoch and the Search for Human Good.* Chicago: Chicago University Press.

Titmuss, R. (1970) *The Gift Relationship.* London: Penguin.

Tonigan, J., Toscova, R., and Connors, G. (2003) 'Spirituality and the Twelve Step Programs: A Guide for Clinicians.' In W. Miller (ed.) *Integrating Spirituality into Treatment.* Washington: American Psychological Association.

Tschudin, V. (2003) *Ethics in Nursing* (3rd edn). London: Butterworth.

UKCC (1992) *Requirements for Pre-registration Nursing Programmes.* London:UKCC.

UKCC (2000) *Requirements for Pre-registration Nursing Programmes.* London:UKCC.

van der Ven, J. (1996) *Formation of the Moral Self.* Grand Rapids: Eerdmans.

van Hooft, S. (1998) 'The Meaning of Suffering.' *Hastings Center Report.* September–October, 13–19.

Vanier, J. (1999) *Becoming Human.* London: Darton, Longman and Todd.

Vanstone, W.H. (1977) *Love's Endeavour, Love's Expense.* London: Darton, Longman and Todd.

Voltaire (1959) *Candide ou l'optimisme.* Paris: Nizet.

Watt, J. (ed.) (1985) *The Church, Medicine and the New Age.* Norwalk: Appleton.

Weil, S. (1977) 'The Love of God and Affliction.' In G. Panichas (ed.) *The Simon Weil Reader.* New York: David McKay Company.

Wilcock, P. (1996) *Spiritual Care of Dying and Bereaved People.* London: SPCK.

Williams, R. (2000) *On Christian Theology.* Oxford: Blackwell.

Williams, R. (2005) 'Faith in the University.' In S. Robinson and C. Katulushi (eds) *Values in Higher Education.* Cardiff: Aureus.

Wilson, L. (1999) *Living Wills.* London: Nursing Times Clinical Monograph.

Woodhead, L. (1992) 'Love and justice.' *Studies in Christian Ethics 5,* 1, 44–61.

Woodhead, L. (1992) 'Feminism and Christian Ethics.' In L. Daly (ed.) *Women's Voices: Essays in Contemporary Feminist Theology.* London: Marshall Pickering.

Wright, S. and Sayre-Adams, J. (2000) *Scared Space.* London: Churchill Livingstone.

Yahne, C. and Miller, W. (2003) 'Evoking Hope.' In W. Miller (ed.) *Integrating Spirituality into Treatment.* Washington: American Psychological Association.

Yorke, M. and Knight, P. (2004) *Embedding employability in the curriculum.* York: LTSN.

Zimbardo, P. (2007) *The Lucifer Effect.* London: Rider.

Subject Index

Author Index